Astro-Guide to Nutrition and Vitamins

Lynne Palmer

Current Printing: 2013

ISBN-10: 0-86690-438-7
ISBN-13: 978-0-86690-438-4

Cover Design: Jack Cipolla

Published by:
American Federation of Astrologers
6535 S. Rural Road
Tempe, AZ 85283

Printed in the United States of America

Books by Lynne Palmer

Money Magic

Your Lucky Days and Numbers

Prosperity Signs

Signs for Success

Astrological Compatibility

Astrological Almanac (annual)

Do-it-Yourself Publicity Directory

Use Astrology and Change your Name

ABC Basic Chart Reading

ABC Chart Erection

ABC Major Progressions

Nixon's Horoscope

Horoscope of Billy Rose

Pluto Ephemeris (1900-2000)

Dedication

I dedicate this book to my friend and client,

Ruth Brown

Grammy and Tony Award winner

and who is in the

Rock and Roll Hall of Fame and

who is a fabulous singer and actress.

Thanks for giving me the idea to write this book,

which will benefit mankind. May God Bless you always.

Cautionary Statement and Disclaimer

The author is an astrologer-writer-reporter, not a doctor. What you do with this information is up to you and not her responsibility.

Warning: This booklet is sold for educational purposes only. Any of the information herein is not medical advice, diagnosis, or prescription. You are warned to seek healing solutions from qualified professionals in the medical profession. Self-treatment can be dangerous if someone is seriously ill.

The author and publisher are not responsible for damage and other liabilities, and cannot guarantee the accuracy, safety, or effectiveness of the data gathered and presented in this work.

Contents

x

Introduction
How to Use This Book

If you want to change your diet, read Chapter One. If you want to detoxify (because Neptune is afflicted and poisons have accumulated), read Chapter Two. If you are interested in taking oxygen-giving supplements, read Chapter Three (these vitamins and minerals help give me tremendous energy). As a preventative against the disease cancer, I take the vitamins and minerals mentioned in Chapter Four (that is, if they are needed, and I can handle them, according to the kinesiology test and whether they are afflicted in my horoscope during a specific time).

On page 101, in Table A, you will notice certain brands and units of measurement given. This table is to make it easy for the chiropractor or nutritionist to test you. When given the kinesiology test, the practitioner has to know how many milligrams or international units are contained in the tablet or capsule. However, if you take a bottle of your choice, it will be listed therein. But can you imagine taking 20 bottles to the tester? If you are going to have this kinesiology test, make a copy of Table A and take it with you. Let the doctor or nutritionist write down beside the vitamin, mineral, or herb, how many a day you can handle. Possibly, you will want to experiment with taking either less than the body can handle or the exact amount.

On page 105, in Table B, find the afflicted planets in your horoscope and on a copy of this worksheet, write the dates that discordant aspects are effective. You can do this for every month, or three or six months, or by the year. How can you tell when a planet is afflicted? The discordant aspects are: semisquare, sesquisquare, square, opposition; the inconjunct, conjunction and parallel become discordant when involved in an aspect with Mars and/or Saturn. Mars and Saturn are the malefic planets. Venus and Jupiter are the benefic planets. The Sun and Moon (luminaries), Mercury, Uranus, Neptune, and Pluto are all neutral.

The secondary progressions (major progressions) indicate when a planet is discordant during a specific time period. This can be ascertained by mathematics or on a computer print out.

Often planets are discordant during a person's entire life. When a planet is afflicted, the body–in my opinion–is depleted in the vitamins that correspond to said planet. Often more than one tablet or capsule is needed. Many years ago, I had a progressed Sun square Mars that was in effect for a year. I went to a chiropractor (Dr. Edwin Samuelson in New York City) and had the kinesiology test. It indicated that I needed 24 kelp tablets a day! I started by taking only a few, but did not feel any better. I gradually worked up to the 24 a day and that is when I felt great! As a result, I always take the maximum amount my body can handle. I find this gives me tremendous energy. Now that I do not have any Sun afflictions, I do not need any kelp tablets!

I have noticed that when I have a discordant transit aspect, I do not need as many supplements as I need when it is a major progressed aspect. However, the slower moving transits are much stronger than an aspect in effect for a day or two with Mercury.

If you are not an astrologer, consult one who can give you the dates when planets are afflicted by major progression. If you can not afford to go to an astrologer, there is an excellent computer service that can send you a print out of your present and future horoscope. Write or call: Astro Numeric Service, PO Box 336 Ashland, OR 97520; 1-627-7464; www.astronumerics.com. Ask for the Hermetic System of progressions. Give them your day, month, year, time and place of birth. Indicate the date you want it to start and for how many years. This service is not free but is economical.

You may not know how to read the computer print-out pages provided by Astro Numeric Service. It is very easy; a child could quickly grasp it. The example is on page 70, Table C, Marla.

On the sample, notice that the planets' names are spelled out except for Merc (Mercury) and Jupi (Jupiter). ASC is the abbreviation for Ascendant, also known as the rising sign or first house cusp. MC is the abbreviation for Media Coeli, also known as the Midheaven or tenth house cusp. If the MC or ASC is afflicted, look up only the planet involved in the aspect with it.

Under *Aspects in Orb* and *Aspects Forming During the Coming Year*, notice the planets and aspects. The aspects are abbreviated:

SSQ Semisquare	CON Conjunction
SQR Square	SSX Semisextile
SQQ Sesquisquare	SXT Sextile
OPP Opposition	TRI Trine
QCX Quincunx	// Parallel

The semisextile, sextile and trine are harmonious aspects. Under *Aspects in Orb*, Marla's Venus Con Neptune is harmonious because it is with a benefic planet, Venus. Marla's ASC Con Saturn (in second column) is discordant because the aspect is with a malefic planet, Saturn. Marla's Saturn (Mars) and Saturn Pluto aspects in the first column under *Aspects in Orb* are discordant parallel aspects because Mars and Saturn are malefic planets.

Under the section *Aspects in Orb*, notice an *Exact* and a *Leave* column. The *Leave* date is when the aspect leaves. The *Exact* date is when the aspect reaches its peak (power, highest point). And after that date it starts getting weaker and becomes less effective as it starts to leave the *Exact* date.

Under *Aspects in Orb*, in the *Exact* column, notice there are lines with no dates listed. This implies that the planet has reached the exact date and on its way out (look in Leave column) or it does not reach the exact date during the time for which the pages were calculated, i.e., if you order three years progressions, then the aspect does not reach an exact date for at least three years from the time your computer print out pages end or even years beyond.

Sometimes an aspect never reaches an exact date. It is in for the duration of your life.

In the example, under *Aspects Forming During the Coming Year*, see the *Enter* date. I ordered Marla's chart on November 18, 1991 (see upper left corner). However, I wanted the aspects to begin January 1, 1991. Therefore, all the aspects that enter from January 1, 1991 to January 1, 1993 (that is, if there are any entering at this time and in this case there were) are given for this three-year report I ordered.

In the example, under *Lunar Aspects*, notice the two columns: *Exact and Aspect*. The starting date for these Moon (lunar) aspects is one month before the exact date. However, there is an exception to this, when months are given. For example:

Exact	*Aspect*
April 6, 1991	// (MC) 7 mo

The preceding implies that the Moon parallel the MC started seven months before April 6, 1991 (April 6, 1991 is the exact date). Parallel aspects often are seen only with the Moon, such as:

Exact	*Aspect*
December 5, 1993	// ASC

This indicates that the aspect (Moon parallel the ASC) began one month before the exact date.

Marla's horoscope under the heading *Aspects Forming During the Coming Year*, second column on page 127, last aspect listed:

Enter	Aspect	Exact	Leave
December 11, 1991	Sun SQR Jupi	1/10/93	---

This reads that on December 11, 1991 a Sun square Jupiter aspect forms and reaches the power point (exact) on January 10, 1993; the leave date is not listed because it goes beyond the time I ordered the chart (beyond the three year progressions). If this were my horoscope, I would read Chapters One (Sun afflicted) and Six (Jupiter afflicted) and go to the chiropractor for a kinesiology test to determine how many of the vitamins and minerals (for the Sun/Jupiter affliction) I could handle. I would start taking them on the December 11, 1991 starting date and would continue to do so until the exact date, January 10, 1993. Also, I would try to eat many of the foods containing these vitamins and minerals, as listed in the Sun and Jupiter chapters.

Good luck! I wish you a healthy future.

Lynne Palmer

Tips and Hints: Foods, Diet

WHEN ONE DOES beneficial things to help others, the immune system is in good shape. Negative emotions, or irritable circumstances block the energy flow and illness is likely to result. Thoughts produce things. In my opinion most illnesses (heart attacks, high blood pressure, etc.) come from the negative thoughts a person carries as well an an improper diet, and a lack of vitamins and minerals. Anger, blaming others, frustrations, worry, depression, etc. are all negative thoughts loaded with electrical charges. When a person becomes egomaniacal, temperamental, frustrated, despondent, worried, excited, pressured, intense, or complaining, he or she creates reversed negative charges that lower his or her electrical output. Thus, not enough oxygenating power is produced to counteract it and a short circuit occurs.

When the oxygen supply is weak, a heart attack or some health problem easily manifests. Those who are happy have better bodily oxygen output and the oxygenation compounds lower blood pressure; better health exists for them than what unhappy people attract. A happy person's bodily conduits have the right connection, polarities and potentials. Thus to avoid any type of disease, change the thoughts from negative to positive.

Vitamins are organic chemical compounds found in foods which, when taken into the body, exercise a profound control over the metabolism. Their presence is required only in minute quantities; health cannot be maintained when certain ones are absent or deficient. Not only is their presence necessary if the endocrine glands are to function properly, but they resemble the hormones secreted by the glands in the body.

The elements found in the average body are calcium, chlorine, carbon, fluorine, hydrogen, iodine, iron, manganese, oxygen, nitrogen, phosphorus, magnesium, silicon, sodium and potassium. All these elements are bountifully supplied in natural foods. However, the manner in which they are prepared can destroy them. It is best to use organic vitamins and minerals instead of inorganic (synthetic) ones. The living organic minerals found in food supplies what the body needs from within, whereas the synthetic vitamins and minerals obtained from the drugstore are ``dead,'' and although they may appear to give energy and be beneficial, they can give neither life nor health. Natural chemicals are needed to keep the body purified and clean.

How many vitamins should be taken daily? How does an individual know whether a vitamin is needed? There is a test - kinesilogy - which is performed by chiropractors and some nutrionists. In my opinion it is the only accurate method to determine the amount that the body needs and can handle at a particular time. When the correct amount of vitamins and minerals are taken, a person feels so much better than when using the ``hit and miss'' method. Note: The horoscope and the kinesiology test may show different deficiencies. When this occurs it indicates that the body cannot at that moment handle that vitamin or mineral. It does not imply it is not needed!

On different days, according to the horoscope, certain vitamins and minerals may be needed that are not needed at other times. When a planet is afflicted in the horoscope, the vitamins and minerals ruled by what that planet needs is what I take to counteract a deficiency. The body is more depleted at that time than at other times, thus requiring a greater input of particular vitamins or minerals.

People get "high" from drinking alcohol because the liquor robs the brain of oxygen. Thus the oxygen-giving supplements may help. I have noticed that Liverall, Vitamin B-12, and Zinc are aids to putting back into the system the B family of vitamins that alcoholic beverages rob from the body. I know people who have taken Liverall or Vitamin B-12 before, after and during drinking alcoholic beverages. When they were taken, especially when the feeling of getting "high" began, the Vitamin B immediately restored the body depletion. Any time the body craves anything, that is a warning that there is a condition of "too much" of something else in the cells. If a person increases the oxygen level with the passing of time, the appetite might be reduced to more normal levels.

If I feel a cold coming, especially the sniffles or a sore throat, I immediately take capsules of red (cayenne) pepper and Vitamin C (rose hips) every hour until it clears. I have known of people who took cayenne pepper capsules and cleared an actual cold within an hour! Also, I refrain from dairy products (it clears colds faster).

Food Combinations

Several different kinds of starches eaten at one meal, tend to cause fermentation (due to their digestive reactions), e.g., potatoes with rice, bread with rice, or bread and potatoes. Protein foods should not be combined with starch foods, e.g., cheese (protein) with bread (starch), frankfurters (protein) and a bun (starch), hamburger (protein) and a bun (starch), meat (protein) and potatoes (starch), fish (protein), and rice (starch). Acid fruits do not combine well with either starches or meat when eaten at the same meal. Spinach eaten at the same meal with other calcium containing foods decreases the amount of calcium assimilated from them, as do cereals unless irradiated or eaten with lettuce, liver or eggs. Note: Fruits should not be eaten at the same meal as protein or starches, e.g., eggs with toast or fruit juice. Two kinds of fruit should not be mixed at a meal. Cane sugar should not be used on fruits. It is best to eat fruits raw. However, applesauce can be beneficial if the entire apple is cooked, including the skin, core (unless wormy) and seeds.

Starchless and Sugarless Vegetables

Lettuce, spinach, all greens (especially dandelion), okra, celery, radishes, string beans, cabbage, cauliflower, brussels sprouts, eggplant, cucumber, zucchini, endive, asparagus, rutabagas, artichokes, turnips and onions are good for the bowels because they furnish bulk.

Sugar Vegetables

Carrots, beets

Carbohydrates (starchy foods)

Bread, pasta, potatoes, flour, grain and wheat products, cereals, beans (navy, lima, butter, kidney, etc), tortillas, rice, green peas, corn, lentils and starchy vegetables—carrots, beets, parsnips. Also ripe fruits, malt, sugar, honey.

Gas-Forming Foods

Beans, cabbage, brussels sprouts, cauliflower, broccoli, onions, green or red peppers, melons, cucumbers and peanuts.

Foods That Relieve Indigestion

Garlic (in any form, raw or capsules which are non-odorous or liquid), acidophilus, cabbage tablets, comfrey-pepsin capsules and chlorodyn capsules. The smooth tasty starches and sweets - new potatoes and young carrots - are the hardest to digest. Note: Acidophilus restores normal flora to the intestinal tract. It helps those with candida (yeast disorders) and is in one's best interest to take when detoxifying, especially when getting a colonic irrigation.

It is not good to eat or drink anything that is very hot or very cold. It is best to stay away from tobacco and chewing gum, and to refrain from eating boiled or fried potatoes (baked with skin is the preferred way to eat potatoes). Never eat a banana unless it is thoroughly ripe (has dark spots and the green on the ends has vanished). Do not drink anything with food: eat it dry so it is thoroughly saturated with saliva in order to alkaline the system. By drinking alcohol and eating food at the same time, an individual does not have the proper power to digest food. Illness could result.

People will most likely gain weight when foods containing fat are eaten. Sugar does not make a person fat. It is fat that makes one fat and fatter. It is fat that causes one to feel sluggish and causes tumors, growths and cysts. Some fats, or lipids, are valuable to the body and are necessary for good health. Oils that come from single sources, such as olive, sunflower, safflower, linseed, canola and corn, are the best for the body. Two tablespoons of oil are needed daily to lubricate the system.

Acid blood is the result of excess sugar and starch. Disease and illness is rare if the blood stream is pure and the body is not full of waste matter and toxins. People who overeat may become ill more quickly than those who eat a little or eat moderately. Overeating makes the stomach, liver, kidneys and bowels work harder. When the food purifies, its poisons are absorbed back into the blood and consequently the entire system is poisoned. Germs cannot live in lemon juice, hydrogen peroxide or an oxygen environment; therefore, be sure the system is properly supplied with them in some form. It is best to try to keep the system alkaline instead of acid. Bread and meat are acid producing foods. They need the alkaline producing vegetables to balance them.

If jewelry, especially rings and copper bracelets, leave a black and blue mark underneath, there is too much acid in the body.

Other Acid Forming Foods

Oysters, chicken, venison, haddock fish, rabbit, veal, lean beef, oatmeal, whole wheat, lean pork, pike fish, eggs, frog meat, fish (in general), crackers, rice, white bread, dried sweet corn, peanuts, coffee and white corn meal.

Alkaline Forming Foods

Figs, potatoes, fruit juices, ginseng root (herb), olives, dried lima beans, spinach, dried beans, raisins, Swiss chard, almonds, parsnips, carrots, dates, beets, celery, bananas, rutabagas (yellow turnips), lettuce, cantaloupe, chestnuts, dried peas, sweet potatoes, dried currants, orange juice, tomatoes, lemons, cauliflower, peaches, pears, watermelon, apples, cabbage, cow's milk, radishes, turnips, onions and asparagus. Note: Starches produce an acid reaction in the body and fruit juices produce an alkaline reaction (the chemical process which takes place after the food enters the body determines acid or alkaline).

Constipating Foods

White bread, white rice, pasta, barley, browned flour gravy, blackberries, boiled milk, hard boiled eggs, meat and cheese.

Foods That Help Prevent Constipation

Greens of all kinds, especially dandelion, tomatoes, asparagus, avocados, cabbage, cauliflower, celery, broccoli, cucumbers, peppers, squash, millet, bran and other fiber grains.

Diet

I believe in eating food, as much as possible, in its raw and natural state. Vegetables should be steamed if they are to be cooked. Some may want to eat two salads a day. I do not eat lettuce; instead I use dandelion greens in my salad (it contains more iron than spinach and more Vitamin A than carrots and has a high cholorphyll content). For salads I use cucumbers, zucchini squash, radishes, Italian parsley and sprouts (sunflower, or a mixture of alfalfa, radish, onion and cabbage). It is best not to use vinegar unless it is organic apple cider vinegar; instead use lime or lemon juice and flax seed oil. In a nutritious diet, plenty of fruit is eaten. However, anyone with diabetes, candida or hypoglycemia can tolerate only grapefruit because it does not contain sugar. Nut butters (almonds and black walnuts) contain iron. Peanuts should be avoided in all forms; they have a fungi and can be a problem for those with candida and many doctors believe they contain carcinogens. Nuts themselves are hard to digest and too many at one time could cause painful gas pockets to form in the colon; therefore, I believe the nut butters are the best. Nuts should not be roasted because the roasting process ruins the oil contained in the nut. It is best to eat them in their raw state.

Avoid junk foods. They are devitamized and can cause illness and poisons. Read labels on products. Avoid junk cereals (with sugar, honey, additives, sweeteners, etc.), candy, soft drinks, sodas, colas, cocoa, doughnuts, sweet rolls, pretzels, potato and corn chips, noodles, crackers, cakes, pie, hamburgers, hot dogs, fried or greasy foods, ice cream, desserts, pastries, coffee and chocolate (the caffeine robs the body of calcium) tea (those that contain caffeine), foods which contain pork, polished white rice, white flour products, white sugar, refined cane sugar and products containing them as well as corn starch, corn syrup, corn sugar, corn breakfast food (cereals); macaroni, corn and cottonseed oil, lard and lard substitutes, stuffed olives, pickles, black pepper (instead use red cayenne pepper), mustard, condiments, spices, salts, salted meat, fish, tabasco sauce, Worcestershire sauce, gravies, liquor. Note: Instead of drinking caffeine products, drink peppermint tea, a natural stimulant. For something sweet try dates, figs and raisins, especially those from health food stores.

Pumpkin and sunflower seeds are good to snack on instead of potato chips and similar foods.

Refined white sugar drains all the mineral salts from the blood, bones and tissues. Junk foods (processed) lose hydrogen peroxide, causing a loss of oxygen, which is vital to maintain life. To replace sugar, use a sweetener such as Equal or Nutra Sweet (these contain aspartic acid and the amino acid phenylalanine, found in protein); when combined they are very sweet. However, they cannot be uses in baking because the high heat for long periods of time causes chemical changes in the amino acids and the loss of the sweet taste; instead, use liquid saccharin in small quantities when baking (this can be hazardous to health so use it sparingly).

Supplements for Extra Energy

Protesoy protein powder or tablets, sold at health food stores, Vitamin C (rose hips), chlorophyll capsules, Liverall capsules, B-12 capsules, chlorella tablets, Vitamin E, bee pollen, cayenne red pepper, Prometol (concentrated wheat germ oil–octacoasanal), ginseng (not for those with hypoglycemia because it stimulates the adrenal glands which can throw sugar in the system). Note: If an individual is getting the proper nutrition through correct eating habits and taking vitamin and mineral supplements, and is then detoxed, it is possible that supplements for extra energy will not be needed. Usually it is when the body is full of poisons that a person feels he or she needs these extra energy boosters. However, if there are few aspects in the horoscope (not much planetary energy, especially with the Sun, Mars and/or Pluto), then these extra energy supplements may be needed.

Suggested Reading

Stellar Healing by C.C. Zain, published by the Church of Light.

Detoxifying

I**T IS IMPORTANT** that the bowels move freely. If they are not completely evacuated at least two or three times a day, constipation results. Every time food is eaten, eight hours later that food should be evacuated through the bowels; otherwise, there is something wrong with the system, and constipation is probably the answer. Carbohydrates, grains and fiber help the body eliminate easily. Millet is the best grain (not many calories, good source of protein, energy-giving, keeps body alkaline). Wheat, brown rice, barley, oats, corn and legumes are also good. (Those with hypoglycemia may find that millet is all they can tolerate because the others contain too much glucose). Whole grains cleanse the body and help keep you fat free. Other foods that cleanse the body are cucumbers, radishes, garlic, onions, okra, spinach, celery, carrots, parsley, tomatoes, asparagus, lettuce, eggplant, ginger root, red and green raw cabbage, broccoli, wheat germ, olive oil and yogurt.

Laxative Foods

Prunes, dates, figs, oranges, apples, bananas, pears, peaches, grapes, grapefruit, watermelon, lemons, raisins, bran, whole-wheat bread, spinach, celery, millet, dandelion greens, lettuce, okra, onions, buttermilk, agar-agar, turnips, squash, parsnips, carrots, olives, olive oil, walnuts, butternuts, cauliflower, pumpkin, blueberries, cherries. Note: those who have diabetes or hypoglycemia may find that raisins, dates, figs, carrots and beets contain too much natural sugar. (Most breads have sugar or honey which also may be difficult to tolerate; however, there are crisp breads made without any form of sugar or yeast content.)

The way I can tell (without looking at my horoscope) that I have poisons in my system is: dizziness, sleepiness, tiredness and the need to take naps. Daily, I use various herbs to detox but when I want to detox in a big way there are various methods to use.

I strongly believe in colonics and have seen unbelievable results take place, not only with myself but with others. Diseases like colitis and cancer have been aided, along with a diet change.

Many people, before they begin to eliminate poisons, cleanse the system by taking an herbal laxative. This will rid the body of much waste matter and mucus, and prevents stirring up of poisons. Inner Clean Herbal Laxative tablets are my choice. Other body purifiers are garlic, aloe vera juice or gel, Vitamin C (rose hips), Colon "8" (Ion Performance brand caplets), chlorophyll capsules, wheat grass and the following herbs for detoxifying: dandelion, chickweed, red clover, bittersweet, cayenne, blue cohosh, St. John's wort, sassafras, parsley—these can be used separately in capsule form or as a beverage (tea). If taken in capsule form, take on an empty stomach before meals, and mix dandelion, chickweed, echinacea and thisilyn together. And before retiring for the night, take Golden Seal herbal capsule. As a tea, different herbs can be mixed (one teaspoon of each to one cup of water for each) and steeped in boiled water for 25 minutes (pour water over herbs); drink this mixture many times throughout the day and night. I always take Golden Seal separately. Also Colon Cleanser (available at health food stores) is good for cleansing the body of poisons.

If a juice machine is available, consider trying this mixture: parsley, cucumber, carrot, celery, spinach, zucchini squash. Do not peel because the vitamins are next to the skin.

I drink aloe vera juice and/or gel many times during the day and evening—in a small amount of water and in between meals.

Note: When detoxing, acidophilus capsules, liquid or tablets keep the normal flora of the intestinal tract in good shape and restores it. Keep the system alkaline; avoid acid forming foods.

There is a purge that can be taken upon rising: 1 tablespoon Epsom Salts dissolved in a half glass of distilled water. Repeat three times in 30 minute intervals. Beginning two hours after the last one, drink one glass of the following mixture every hour: 12 oranges (do not use if diabetic or hypoglycemic), juice of 6 fresh lemons, 6 grapefruit. Store in a gallon glass jar and fill with distilled water. Do not eat during the day; in the evening eat an orange or grapefruit. Note: If you are diabetic or hypoglycemic, do not fast unless your physician has given you permission to do so.

There is a 10-day Colon Cleanse kit produced by Aerobic Life Products. It is said that this is an unbelievable way to rid the body of waste matter that has been fermenting for years. Within three days, garbage comes flowing out–sometimes two feet or more. This does not upset the normal absorption of minerals that go back through the colon into the blood.

The blood stream becomes cleansed when a lot of grape, orange, apple or grapefruit juice is consumed. The larger the intake, the quicker the body is cleansed. Water should be drunk between meals, not with meals. A large raw vegetable salad helps in the cleansing process. Note: Do not mix the fruit juices; drink different ones at different intervals. Do not put any sweetener on any fruits. If fruit is not ripe before picking, it will not be as effective in the cleansing. Eat fruits and vegetables, and eliminate starches, oils, butter, sugar, canned fruits and vegetables, eggs, desserts and all junk food. Vary the fruit, including fresh pineapple, pears, plums, apples, cherries, peaches, strawberries and blueberries. When cleansing the body and taking mineral and vitamin supplements, the body is being fed through the blood, giving it the proper nutrition needed. Eat fresh fruits and vegetables in large quantities to prevent wrinkles and the shrinking of the stomach and intestines. Do not eat sugar or protein during the cleansing time because they, as well as starches, tend to clog the system and may be difficult to digest. This cleansing program may be followed for several days or a week. Once finished, return to other foods but eat sparingly and do not eat junk foods.

The five organs that eliminate poisons are liver, kidneys, bowels, lungs and skin.

To Detox the Kidneys

One lemon in a cup of hot water once a day mid-morning.

To Detox the Lungs

Avoid mucous forming foods (milk, cheese, yogurt, ice cream, etc.). In the morning upon arising, sniff water in the nose, blow it out. Repeat several times. Do deep breathing for 12 minutes, and take moderate exercise, especially in the open air.

To Detox the Liver

Upon rising, mix the juice from one-half squeezed lemon, 1 teaspoon cold pressed olive oil and 6 ounces warm water; sip slowly and do not eat for an hour. Also take Thisilyn herb capsule on an empty stomach and/or Thioctic (Thiox).

To Detox the Bowels (Colon)

Colon cleanser, Herbal Laxative tablets, colonics, aloe vera juice or gel, Colon "8", Vitamin C, chlorophyll, dandelion, chickweed, or golden seal herb capsules (the products mentioned in this chapter under laxative foods), as well as fruits and vegetables as a diet, or the "purge" (see page 9).

To Detox the Skin

The skin eliminates poisons only when wet; therefore, daily baths help. Take a hot shower in the morning. Sit in a tub of water with one cup apple cider vinegar added to it, and afterwards rub the skin briskly with a towel until a warn glow is felt. Or take a bath with Epson salts (three pounds to a tub filled with water). Drink plenty of water or broth while in the tub, and massage the body with a loofah dipped in Epson salt water. This action increases the activity of the skin and the circulation. Finish with a cool shower and, when drying, rub the body vigorously until a warm glow is felt.

Oxygen-Giving Supplements

HYDROGEN AND OXYGEN are two gases necessary for life. When combined with carbon and nitrogen they form proteins; when combined with carbon they form carbohydrates; when combined with each other, they make water, and if water is saturated with extra oxygen, it results hydrogen peroxide. All these elements and compounds exist in our blood.

Oxygen is a dissolver and is found everywhere in the air, fruits and vegetables. When blood passes through the lungs, it is purified by oxygen. Everyone needs more oxygen because it hastens elimination and burns poisons. Oxygen keeps cells flexible and clean, and removes unneeded structure. The hydrogen gives our bodies structure and the oxygen burns the food that is used to make the structure, as well as cleaning up afterwards. Oxidation is a process of delivering nutrients, digesting food and releasing energy. Oxygen can slow the aging process by keeping cells clean so that they wear out slowly.

Lack of oxygen and minerals in the vital fluids (lack of health maintaining oxidation) is the main cause of disease. The digestive tract must be clean for the active oxygen to reach and pass through the capillaries and blood vessels, which help rid the body of poison (garbage). To avoid disease the bowels should be clean (free from obstruction as well as old fecal matter) so that oxygen and organic minerals can get through. When food rots inside the body instead of being absorbed back into the blood, its absorptive work and increasing purification are stopped; body fluids, the lymph and the blood are always dirty and thus do not function well or for long. Therefore, it is important to get oxygen-giving substances into the system.

Disease germs cannot live in a high oxygen environment. If there is not enough oxygen, then both the solidifying functions and incomplete combustion occur to excess. Residual, incomplete combustion byproducts collect in the cells. Then the body is toxic, or has a buildup of waste products. Under these conditions the immune system has a hard time fighting off disease. If the body's oxygen level drops too low, energy is low. Illness might result if the immune system cannot clean up the dirt from the system.

Hydrogen peroxide keeps the body germ and bacteria free. The hydrogen peroxides and other free radical scavengers created by blood ozonation identify and destroy diseased cells. Repeated ozone application destroys them. Cells inflicted with a virus have a weakened vitality which shows up as lowered levels of enzyme activity. A free radical hydrogen peroxide sees the low enzyme level of the diseased cells as a threat to the body's well being and attacks them. Both are destroyed in the process, which benefits the person so afflicted.

Minerals are the basic building blocks of the body and are vital to oxygenation. Fluoride reduces the body's ability to oxygenate. Oxygen intake into the system is an enzyme reaction and fluoride stops enzymes. This is a low grade poisoning which stops beneath the surface in most people, but in those whose health is on the decline it produces illness.

Cancer and AIDS cannot grow in an oxygen environment. In fact, cancer cells are "anaerobic" and they function without oxygen. Oxygen destroys "anaerobic" bacteria and "anaerobic" cells. Ozone, oxygen and hydrogen peroxide help restore kidney functions and hair loss, and are beneficial for those who suffer with high blood pressure, arthritis, multiple sclerosis, acne, candida, diabetes, heart problems, hepatitis, herpes, leukemia, ulcers, the flue, or colds. Oxygen, ozone and hydrogen peroxide dissolve cholesterol, plaque and triglycerides. Also, they have a positive effect on problems with sinuses, mouth diseases, bunions and other foot ailments.

AIDS is a virus and a virus works by burrowing in and attaching itself to a cell's genetic material. It is difficult to eradicate inside the cells, without killing everything else in the process. However, doctors in Germany (one is Dr. Horst Kief) have been able to cure patients of AIDS by using ozone, oxygen and hydrogen peroxide, without damage to the cells, organs or body. This treatment takes from five days to a month and the patient is sent home and often cured or partially cured.

Exercise gets oxygen into the body so that it feels refreshed. Most people have a build-up of waste products in their cells, do not exercise enough, eat junk food and have shortness of breath. They are not getting enough oxygen and need to do deep breathing exercises, as well as change the diet.

Eating foods which contain the essential polyunsaturated fatty acids enhances oxygenation. These fatty acids can be found naturally in carotene, saffron and flaxseed oil. Anything that is eaten that is hydrogenated defeats the purpose of oxygenation. A good example is margarine, which is oil with hydrogen bubbled through it. Also, fried food defeats oxygenation. The best oil for human consumption is fresh flaxseed oil; the best brand which is not rancid (like some) is spectrum Naturals "Veg-Omega-3 Certified Organic Flax Oil." Never heat it or its benefits will be destroyed. If the taste is unpleasant, mix it with cold pressed olive oil and use as salad dressing. If it is necessary to cook in an oil, use sunflower oil because when heat is applied to it, the cancer causing agents are not produced as they are with butter or other oils.

Natural hydrogen peroxide is found in sea water, salt, grapefruit, apples, watermelons, raw potatoes, cabbage, asparagus, green peppers, watercress, aloe vera juice or gel, rainwater, raw green vegetables, Perrier water, raw comb honey, egg yolks, liver (calf, pork), sprouts, fresh squeezed orange juice, and these oxygen-giving supplements: Sod, Germanium, Laetrile (B-17), Octacosanol, Co-enzyme Q-10, Vitamins A, C, E and F, Selenium (it must be taken with Vitamin E to be oxygen-giving), Chlorophyll and Ginseng Root (chew its root or drink its extracts and oxygenation is increased; it contains a lot of chlorophyll and alkalines the system).

The Fountain of Youth

Aloe vera juice and oxygen-giving vitamins will help maintain youth and the absence of wrinkles. Aging occurs when sugar and junk foods are eaten. Skin looks vibrant with the right diet, vitamins and minerals.

The best form of oxygen, also a benefit to anti-aging, is Cell Food, which is made from natural plant substances. It contains dissolved oxygen, 78 ionic-collodial and 34 minerals of trace minerals and elements, 34 enzymes, 17 amino acids and electrolytes. The dissolved oxygen and other ingredients come from the clean Southern Seas surrounding New Zealand. It gives immediate energy and gets oxygen to the cells of the body.

The Disease Cancer

THE AFFLICTED PLANETS in a person's horoscope that give a predisposition for the disease cancer are Mars (protein metabolism problem), Jupiter (liver, fats, growths), Saturn (salt mineral deficiencies, negativity, weight loss), Neptune (poisons, fluids) and Pluto (protein metabolism problem). For more detail regarding these planets and their corresponding vitamins and minerals, refer to each planet's section in Part Two.

The underlying cause for cancer development is the diseased condition of the liver. It may not show up for years because the liver does not present any characteristic symptoms of pain for a long time, even years. Thus cancer can be a hidden disease until symptoms of one or several growths appear and are discovered.

Cancer cells always show an absence of Vitamins A, B and C, and oxidation substances. Vitamin A is important because its presence brings about the decomposition of certain fatty acids. The process of Vitamin C is of utmost importance in the entire oxidation process that takes place in the cells. Vitamin B, along with Vitamin C, may increase twice or even threefold the oxidating enzymes in the blood, which are important to the whole oxidation process.

Salt causes increased cramping of the capillaries and has been known to be concentrated in body cells which become increasingly cancerous. To help prevent cancer, avoid junk foods such as refined, canned, bottled, powdered and frozen food with artificial coloring (used in food processing, it is cancer producing and impairs and destroys oxidation-enzymes) or preservatives. Eat no dairy products or food with nitrates (used in smoked meats, ham, back, sausage, turkey, fish) or white bread, sugar or flour (they cause a deficiency in Vitamin B-1). Stay away from refined and processed oils, a high consumption of salt (sodium destroys the potassium in the system), refined carbohydrates (not natural) and chicken and meat (too many hormones injected into them to fatten them up). Do not overeat or drink liquids (soups, beverages) too hot or too cold (the same goes with food). Water at room temperature is best. Quit smoking (arsenic, a poison, is used on tobacco leaves which are later smoked). Avoid fats heated too many times to high temperatures (fried foods, i.e., french fries) because they cause a deficiency in the B vitamins, Vitamin C and the minerals. Note: Refer to page 7 for other junk foods.

To help prevent cancer, use the natural salt which many vegetables contain (i.e., celery) and eat plenty of fruits and vegetables (preferably those with high potassium and low sodium content and especially vegetables that are green–the greener, the better because there is more chlorophyll). Eat plenty of salads and drink apple, carrot, celery and green leafy vegetable juices. Garlic helps retard cancer growth (the whole garlic clove is best). Vegetables that help fight cancer are sprouts, broccoli, mung beans, lentils and wheat grass. Foods which may prevent carcinogenic chemicals (cancer forming) from damaging cellular DNA: strawberries, raspberries, logan berries, grapes, plums and Brazil nuts. Note: Eat mostly (75 percent) raw food because it is more digestible and vitamins and minerals are not lost as they are when cooked.

To help prevent cancer, an individual needs all of the B family of vitamins (especially Vitamin B-1, Choline, Niacin, Folic

The Disease Cancer

Acid, B-12), Vitamins A and C, Chlorophyll, Calcium, Zinc, Phosphorus, Selenium, Beta-Pepsin—hydrochloric acid needed in the stomach to digest Vitamin A), all of the oxygen-giving supplements (refer to Part One/Chapter Three) and all of the vitamins and minerals listed in Part Two under afflicted Mars, Jupiter, Saturn, Neptune and Pluto.

Cancer and Vitamin C

Cancer cells are known to move around in a body because of an inherent propensity which becomes manifest solely because they have lost their connective tissue anchorage as a direct result of a Vitamin C deficiency. Precancerous tissues always show a loss of connective tissue. The cement which holds cells together can be manufactured only if Vitamin C is present in ample quantity.

Easy bruising is one of the earliest symptoms of a Vitamin C deficiency. It may be the first symptom, or a warning, of a predisposition for cancer. Poisons other than nicotine are counteracted by Vitamin C in the body, and the Vitamin C is used immediately when it contacts the poison. When Vitamin C is not present, the connective tissues may be destroyed and lead the way for cancer to spread rapidly through the body. If gums bleed, teeth are loose, bruises occur easily, colds develop readily, open sores heal slowly, or there is exposure to tobacco or smoke, it is important to get Vitamin C into the system because the preceding could mean a deficiency of Vitamin C and a predisposition for cancer.

Sun Afflicted...
Vitamins, Minerals

WHEN THE SUN is afflicted the body needs iodine (found in kelp), manganese, chlorophyll, Vitamin A (carotene is non-toxic), Vitamin B-1, B-2, B-12 (if an allergy exists, perhaps Cracked Cell Chlorella or Liverall—dessicated liver—will be easy to tolerate, Folic Acid (B-9), Niacin (no-flush best), and Co-enzyme Q-10. Note: Cracked Cell Chlorella (the best Chlorella is Cracked Cell) is ocean algae. It is a good source of chlorophyll, iron, Vitamin A and B-2. It is a healing agent and gives one energy. It is incompatible with other forms of chlorophyll; thus, take them 12 hours apart. Also for Sun afflictions (or planets in Leo afflicted), hawthorn, kyolic garlic, grape seed extract and Cell Food.

Vitamin and Mineral Food Sources

Iodine: Asparagus, onions, garlic, artichokes, carrots, peas, dried beans, tomatoes, potato skins, spinach, Swiss chard, fish (especially flounder, haddock), most sea foods (especially oysters, lobster), agar-agar, all garden vegetables, iodized salt (however kelp or seaweed in dried form is best).

Manganese: Green vegetables, string beans, kale, dandelion greens, senna and peppermint leaves, parsley, endive, lettuce, mustard greens, cucumbers, fruits, egg yolks, legumes, whole grains, whole wheat, almonds, walnuts, raspberries, dates, celery, tomatoes, green papers, chestnuts, bananas, watercress, huckleberries, oatmeal, onions, beets, rhubarb.

Chlorophyll: The oxidation-enzymes (oxygen-giving) found only in green leafy vegetables especially dandelion, spinach, mustard greens.

Vitamin A (Carotene): Milk, cream, butter, cream cheese, eggs, bananas, carrots, asparagus, fish liver oil, most dairy products (including milk), yellow and green fruits and vegetables, parsley, spinach, kale, lettuce, dandelion, cheese, beef liver (also pork, calf, and lamb liver), yellow corn, okra, string beans, watercress, avocado, mangoes, papayas, peaches, pineapple, oranges, hubbard squash, summer squash, beef and lamb kidney, dried prunes, halibut, cod and salmon liver oils. escarole, broccoli, swiss chard, cantaloupe, mustard greens, pumpkin, apricots, beets, endive, parsnips, peas, alfalfa leaf meal, dried peaches, red and green peppers, yellow squash (crookneck), zucchini squash, sweet potatoes, yams, tomatoes, turnip greens.

Vitamin B-1: Wheat germ, brewer's yeast (the best source of B1), liver, whole grains, oatmeal, rolled oats, peanuts, nuts fish, poultry, beans, meat, whole wheat bread, whole cereals, rice polishings (not refined; brown natural is the best source), soy beans, pork ham, pecans, beef heart, hazel nuts, lentils, lima beans, rye, walnuts, green peas, dry navy beans, egg yolks, dried skim milk, white corn meal.

Vitamin B-5: Soybeans, organ meats, brewer's yeast, egg yolks, whole grain cereals, legumes, red kidney beans.

Vitamin B-12: Liver, organ meats, eggs, milk, fish cheese.

Vitamin B-15: Brewers yeast, brown rice, whole grains, pumpkin, and sesame seeds.

Folic Acid (a B Vitamin): Fruits, tomatoes, green leafy vegetables, organ meats, brewer's yeast, milk products, spinach, asparagus, green beans.

Niacin (a B Vitamin): Brewer's yeast, meat, poultry, fish, milk products, peanuts, corn meal. Note: when taking brewer's yeast, it is preferable to take it in powder form because it would take an enormous amount of tablets to equal the strength of a few tablespoons of the powder form. Bran is a rich source of the B family of vitamins; it relieves constipation because of the large amount of cellulose it contains.

Co-enzyme Q-10: Mackerel, sardines, cereals (especially bran), nuts, dark green vegetables (dandelion, spinach, broccoli), soy beans, soy and sesame oils.

Vitamin and Mineral Functions

Iodine: Component of hormone thyroxine which controls metabolism. The thyroid, through the hormone thyroxine, determines growth, controls body temperature, regulates the metabolism or the burning of food in the body, and influences, to a great extent, mental and emotional balance. Also, it is of special importance for the proper functioning of the reproductive system. Disorders of the thyroid gland are apparently caused by two conditions: 1) When there is a lack of sufficient iodine in the diet, the thyroid cannot obtain enough to manufacture thyroxine; and 2) a disorder of the body which creates a demand for much more thyroxine than the gland can manufacture and, therefore, more iodine than is available in the diet. It is best to make sure that the thyroid gland has enough iodine to manufacture thyroxine naturally; thus, foods and supplements containing iodine are beneficial.

Manganese: A strong purifier and effective neutralizer of body acids. Also it is an enzyme activator, helps carbohydrate, fat, and sex hormone production, and skeletal development.

Chlorophyll: All living things require oxygen which, by the process of oxidation, changes food into energy and growth. This process is aided by the presence of chlorophyll. Foods containing chlorophyll give energy and vitality and, without chlorophyll, the body is impoverished. Chlorophyll cleanses the body and gives it life.

Vitamin A (Carotene): The presence of Vitamin A is of utmost importance in the entire oxidation process that takes place in cells. It strengthens the respiratory tract's delicate tissues against bacterial invaders. It keeps the mucous lining of the digestive tract in healthy condition (also needed is B-1, B-2 and C). Vitamin A may affect the lining of the gall bladder. It is important to the health of all the membranes of the body, but especially the linings of organs and passageways. It protects the epithelial tissue. It is needed in normal cell growth and development. It is for the growth and repair of body tissues (resist infection), bone and tooth formation, visual purple production (necessary for night vision). Vitamin A brings about the decomposition of certain fatty acids; therefore, its presence is necessary. It is protective against infection by providing for the health of the mucous membranes, which germs attack. Exercise causes Vitamin A to be absorbed by the body. For the proper use of Vitamin A in the body, Vitamin C and D are needed simultaneously. If Vitamin E is not present, Vitamin A is quickly used up by oxygen. Vitamin A is fat soluble, hence oils and fats favor its absorption. However, carotene is water soluble and does not cause toxic conditions when taken to excess; but Vitamin A causes toxic conditions when taken in abundance. Carotene is in many fruits and vegetables and is converted into Vitamin A in the body-the same goes with Carotene supplements. Mineral oil prevents absorption of Vitamin A.

Vitamin B-1: It is needed every moment in the mucous lining of the digestive tract whenever carbohydrates of any kind are eaten. It is an essential part of the enzyme system, necessary for breaking down carbohydrates into easily digestive substances. It is for the nerves and brain, appetite maintenance, growth, muscle tone, nerve function and digestion.

Vitamin B-5: It converts nutrients into energy, is involved in the formation of some fats and is needed for vitamin utilization.

Vitamin B-12: It is needed for carbohydrate, fat and protein metabolism, maintains a healthy nervous system and is good for blood cell formation and pernicious anemia.

Vitamin B-15: It is for the metabolism of sugar, fats and proteins, and stimulates the nerve and glandular systems. It is needed for cell respiration.

Folic Acid: It is needed for red blood cell formation, protein metabolism, growth and cell division.

Niacin: It is needed for healthy gums and blood circulation, and for fat, carbohydrate and protein metabolism. Also it is the health of the skin, tongue and digestive system. It occurs in living cells as an essential substance for growth.

Co-enzyme Q-10: It strengthens the immune system and is oxygen-giving and protects the cells against free radicals that threaten the cells' oxygen supply. It increases the production of antibodies. It decreases reduction in size and quantity of tumors and lowers cancer mortality. Every cell in the body has co-enzyme Q-10 in it. It has the ability to transfer electrons as needed from molecule to molecule. The human body will not function without it and can get it from food. It supplies quick energy to the cells and is the igniting spark and nutrient that permits energy production. Without it there is no respiration and thus no life. If the cells are in good shape, they are oxygenating; if not, only some are oxygenating.

B Family of Vitamins in General: The central nervous system provides the greatest means for storage of the B family of vitamins in the body; storage of B vitamins in all other parts of the body is more rapidly exhausted on a diet void of Vitamin B. Mental exertion depletes the storage in the brain while physical exertion reduces the reserves in the spinal motor nerves. This is based on the assumption that the nerve cells of the brain and spinal cord provide vitamin storage in much the same way a battery stores electricity; mental and physical activity discharge the storage, while sleep and rest effect recharge. There is little storage of excess Vitamin B in the body and deficiency symptoms occur within a few days after withdrawal of the vitamin source. Vitamin B is effective against invading germs. All of the B vitamins improve the action of the liver. The B vitamins relieve frequent constipation. They are absolutely necessary for the proper use of carbohydrates by the body. A diet high in refined carbohydrates (white sugar, white flour, and bread) is automatically low in minerals and vitamins, as well as the cellulose needed to assure the proper working of the digestive tract. Anyone eating a high carbohydrate diet automatically has an increased need for B Vitamins. Anyone who is easily fatigued or chilled or has an infection, fever or fear (worry) needs to increase the B vitamins. Vitamin B is necessary to accompany the carbohydrates through the digestive tract.

Vitamin and Mineral Deficiency Symptoms

Iodine: A thyroid problem, goiter, dry skin and hair, nervousness, obesity. There is a relationship between goiter and too much cyanide in food or water. Organic cyanide is present in "trace" amounts in cabbage, peas, lentils, soybeans, mustard seed and peanuts. If eaten in large quantities to the exclusion of all other foods, a goiter could develop; therefore, eat them in small amounts.

Manganese: Dizziness, ear noises, and poor muscle coordination are the deficiency symptoms.

Chlorophyll: Cooking foods results in a deficiency of chlorophyll (the substance that makes plants green) and consequently a deficiency occurs in all the products which chlorophyll assists in manufacturing in the body. If little or no chlorophyll is present, these oxidation enzymes cannot do their job. The result, therefore, is an impoverishment of the organism in the vital oxidation enzymes and in the vitamins, especially Vitamin C. Thus the deficiency impairs the vital forces (shuts them down), soon inertia and a lack of energy are felt.

Vitamin A (Carotene): A deficiency of Vitamin A shows up first in a sloughing off of the cells which line the digestive, respiratory and reproductive tracts. This indicates a weakness of the cells which make up the structure of these important organs, and serves as a warning that nutrition to these parts is lacking. Its deficiency lowers resistance to infection and tends to prolong colds, encourages the skin to get dry and scaly and lose its sensitivity to touch, promotes the improper formation and maintenance of tooth enamel, decreases the ability to see in dim light and adjust vision quickly after glare, causes the inability to nourish a fetus in the uterus, and causes development of bladder stone.

Lack of Vitamin A disorders the function of the pituitary gland. The pituitary gland secrets a substance which regulates the thyroid. Lacking Vitamin A, this entire process goes awry. Also, its deficiency is responsible for hardening and roughening of the skin, night blindness and degeneration of mucous membranes. Ironically, those who suffer from night blindness also suffer from goiter because both a lack Vitamin A in the diet.

A Vitamin A deficiency affects the spinal cord and nervous system. This makes it easier for bacteria to enter the deeper layers of the skin and nerves, thus lowering the body's resistance to infection. Vitamin A is necessary for the normal cellular metabolism of the body. The nerves are affected by its deficiency and it has a connection with polio. A lack of Vitamin A leads to structural changes affecting the skin. When there are severe infections, Vitamin A is used up so rapidly by body tissues that there is never enough left over for ordinary functions. The frequency of liver disorder in arthritics suggests that the liver might be unable to do its work of transforming Carotene into Vitamin A. Cancer of the reproductive organs can result from lack of Vitamin A, in many cases caused by faulty absorption of Vitamin A due to lack of hydrochloric acid in the stomach. A loss of smell and appetite, and susceptibility to infection, tooth decay and frequent fatigue are some more of Vitamin A's deficiency symptoms. The need for Vitamin A increases greatly in fevers and lowers resistance to disease.

Vitamin B-1: A lack may begin to operate by damaging the liver; however slight it may be, it may be enough to keep the liver from activating female hormones, which is one of its functions. Thus, material might accumulate in the body and cause cancer of the uterus.

A lack of Vitamin B-1 can change the entire digestive tract and produce many and varied stomach disorders. There is a loss of appetite, fatigue and the stomach and intestines cannot contract normally because food is not well mixed with digestive enzymes. The muscles of the stomach and intestines function poorly; thus, constipation can occur easily. Often there is a loss of weight, vomiting, backache, sore muscles, numbness, burning feet, mental depression and headaches. Hydrochloric acid decreases as well as the flow of digestive juices from the pancreas and gall bladder.

A lack of Vitamin B-1 can cause nerve disorders, nervousness and anorexia nervosa, and can be dangerous to life. It can cause memory defects, disorientation, confusion, periods of excitement, depression, mania, delirium, paranoia and mental illness, and may bring on neuritis or beri-beri. In the eyes it could take the form of retrobulbar neuritis (pains behind the eyeball). Its deficiency may cause heart irregularity or hardening of the arteries. Tobacco and alcohol decrease Vitamin B-1; thus the body requirement of it increases.

It may cause chronic fatigue and certain kinds of deafness due to a nerve disturbance. Deposits of cholesterol collecting in the walls of the tiny blood vessels may have a lot to do with this kind of deafness.

A Vitamin B-1 deficiency can cause low blood pressure, making a person feel weak, tired, dizzy, lightheaded or faint regardless of whether lying down, standing or sitting up. The individual may act grouchy, feel inefficient or be sleepless. A diet low in protein makes one prone to eat more starchy and sugary foods. The more starches and sweets eaten, the more Vitamin B-1 the body needs.

If the carbohydrates eaten are beans, potatoes, bananas, nuts, peas and other natural foods, then the body is getting plenty of Vitamin B-1 and Niacin, which assures it of being able to digest the starches. If, however, the diet consists of refined carbohydrates (white flour, white sugar), cereals (processed), bakery products, candy, ice cream, soft drinks, cakes, pies, or other starchy or sugary foods made of refined products, the individual is heading for indigestion and a Vitamin B-1 deficiency because this vitamin and Niacin have been removed from these refined products.

No refined sugar can give energy unless Vitamin B-1 is present to break it down from pyruvic acid to energy, carbon dioxide and water. It is present in natural foods and therefore the body does not have difficulty in breaking it down in the system. When white sugar products are eaten, or drunk in coffee, the digestive tract is presented with large quantities of sugar to be digested; thus there is no Vitamin B-1 can handle the job. In order for the body to handle this sugar at all, it must steal Vitamin B-1 from other processes and from its storage place in the liver, kidney and heart. Therefore, if white sugar is eaten on a daily basis, the body probably will suffer from a deficiency in Vitamin B-1. If there is a heart problem, such a dietary habit is cold suicide. A lack of Vitamin B-1 impairs the function of the heart, increases the tendency to extravascular fluid collection and results in terminal cardiac standstill. Brewer's yeast, desiccated liver and wheat germ supplements may help prevent undue accumulation of fatty deposits in the artery walls. Vitamin B-1 is used in the process by which the body uses fat.

Vitamin B-5: Its deficiency symptoms are vomiting, stomach stress, restlessness, infections and muscle cramps.

Vitamin B-12: Its deficiency symptoms are nervousness (not connected with the mind). They include ``pins and needles" sensations, numbness, stiffness, feelings of hot and cold, local feelings of deadness, tightness and shooting pains, fatigue, brain degeneration, neuritis, pernicious anemia, and mental confusion. People who lack hydrochloric acid (a digestive juice) in their stomachs, digest Vitamin B-12 poorly.

Vitamin B-15: A lack of this vitamin could cause heart disease, glandular and nervous disorders, and impaired circulation.

Folic Acid: Its lack causes anemia, graying hair, poor growth, and gastrointestinal troubles.

Niacin: It's lack causes general fatigue, indigestion, irritability, loss of appetite, skin disorders, digestive disorders, nervousness. Involved in pellagra (a chronic disease with skin disruptions, digestive and nervous disturbances, and eventual mental deterioration), psoriasis (skin eruptions). Note: a lack of niacin over a long period may result in a decrease of hydrochloric acid (an important digestive juice) in the stomach, which will lead to further indigestion.

Co-enzyme Q-10: Its lack may possibly accelerate aging, whereas an increase of it keeps one young. As the body ages, especially after the age of 35, the liver may not be able to produce or convert it as it did previously; thus, it's easy to become deficient in Co-enzyme Q-10.

B Family of Vitamins in General: The storage of Vitamin B in the body is very limited. There is an increased bodily demand for Vitamin B with fever or increased physical exertion. When a great thirst is satisifed, the B vitamins and Vitamin C are washed out. Sugar and white flour rob the body of B vitamins.

Since digestive disturbances are unusually associated with beri-beri, poliomyelitis and encephalitis, the depletion of the nerve-protective B vitamins is not only hastened, but the intake of new supplies is impeded; therefore, there is a severe Vitamin B deficiency in these cases. Many diseases of the nervous system are associated with a Vitamin B deficiency.

In cases of cancer the B Vitamins destroy the excess estrogenic and androgenic hormones faster, thus cutting down the excess stimulation to breast and prostate cancer. Arthritics have difficulty assimilating carbohydrates (sugars and starches); thus a Vitamin B deficiency occurs. The B Vitamins are involved in eye health - B-2, B-5, B-6, Niacin and Folic Acid are important for healthy eyes. Alcoholics need more B vitamins than the average person because alcohol uses up Vitamin B.

A lack of B vitamins may create fatigue, apathy, muscle and joint pains, lack of appetite, constipation, fragile fingernails (easily broken and with ridges extending lengthwise or horizontally). The stomach and intestines are relaxed and sluggish with a Vitamin B deficiency.

Vitamin and Mineral Therapeutic Applications

Iodine: Goiter, hair problems, atherosclerosis and hyperthyroidism; may be effective as a cure or be a preventive against polio. Note: some iodine is lost in perspiration, which occurs most frequently in summer (hot) months (when most polio cases occur). Also in summer thyroid gland secretions are the lowest, thus resulting in less iodine available to the body.

Manganese: Diabetes, loss of coordination and muscle strength, and multiple sclerosis.

Chlorophyll: Prevents cataracts.

Vitamin A: Bronchial asthma, colds, migraine, infections, glaucoma, emphysema, acne, boils, allergies, tooth and gum disorders, pneumonia, prostrate trouble, gall bladder problems, and those who have hearing defects have been helped.

Vitamin B-1: Improved heart function, indigestion, nausea, constipation, alleviates pain, rapid heart rate.

Vitamin B-5: Digestive disorders, stress, fatigue, infections, arthritis.

Vitamin B-12: Stress, fatigue, mild memory loss, insomnia, anemia, depression, lack of concentration, shingles, inflammatory skin diseases, lumbago, osteoarthritis, osteoporosis, psychosis, cerebral (mental) manifestations, vascular diseases, mental illness and night cramps in the legs, and alcoholism.

Vitamin B-15: Alcoholism, asthma, emphysema, atherosclerosis, heart disease, rheumatism and premature aging.

Folic Acid: Anemia, atherosclerosis, leg and stomach ulcers, dropsy, diarrhea, menstrual problems and gray hair.

Niacin: Diarrhea, anemia, high blood pressure, leg cramps, acne, migraines, halitosis, pellagra, chronic alcoholism, senility, and cirrhosis of the liver.

Co-enzyme Q-10: It can accelerate weight loss in some people as it manipulates oxygen. It can increase oxygen levels when necessary and reduce them if they threaten to reach toxic levels. Possibly Co-enzyme Q-10 could be an immune booster and help AIDS. It could be helpful to those who have cancer. It could help prevent heart disease. It removes free radicals. It is an oxygen-giving supplement.

B Family of Vitamins in General: The B vitamins improve the action of the liver, thus ensuring better nutrition for all the tissues of the body. They are good for neuritis and paralysis. The B family of vitamins is beneficial for diabetics who require more B-1, B-2, B-12 and Niacin than does the average healthy person. It is possible they help decrease the insulin requirement and bring about considerable improvement in diabetes.

The Sun

The Sun governs the heart (blood pumped to various parts of the body), the spleen (vital electric energy stored there), and the spine. The action of the two front pituitary hormones and the thyroid gland is influenced by the Sun. One's vitality is ruled by the Sun. The Sun governs the electric energy of the body.

The thyroid is a ductless gland located at the base of the neck. It is an organ of the body which secretes a fluid, but it has no "duct" or opening through which the fluid passes to another part of the body. So the fluid manufactured by the thyroid gland passes directly into the blood stream. This fluid, or hormone thyroxine, is made by the thyroid gland out of iodine and the amino acid tyrosine (amino acids are forms of protein.) The thyroid rules the rate of growth, the rate at which food is burned for energy, emotions, the personality, and the way the body handles cholesterol. The thyroid manufactures its hormone thyroxin from its supply of iodine and tyrosine.

When the supply of iodine is short or interrupted, the thyroid strains itself to make thyroxin, often enlarging until a goiter is formed. The goiter is a swelling (enlargement) of the thyroid gland—a shortage of iodine in the diet. It is possible that the relationship between arteriosclerosis and goiter might be due to underproduction or overproduction of thyroxin stimulated by the pituitary gland. The secretions of the thyroid gland decrease with age, sometimes diminishing to the extent that the body's needs are not met. Also hardening of the arteries may occur when a metabolism failure allows cholesterol to collect in the arteries instead of using or expelling it from the body. The thyroid gland is largely concerned with metabolism.

When the Sun is afflicted in a horoscope thyroxin tends to drive water from the body. A person who has an active thyroid (Sun strong) loses water rapidly; a person who has a sluggish thyroid (Sun afflicted) tends to retain the water he or she drinks. The thyroid is the gland of energy production and when the Sun is discordant in the horoscope there is a depletion of the front pituitary gland's secretion of thyroxin, or oversecretion of thyroxin which causes energy to be used too fast. Thyroxin is poured into the blood stream, and this stimulates the heart and contracts the blood vessels. The vitamins exercise vital control over tissue construction and the production of energy. The Sun rules the life controlling vitamins.

Thyroxin and the front pituitary glands (especially the thyroid) respond with great sensitivity to emotional conditions. The feeling of hurry, or strain, high pressure or worry, or forcing oneself to continue after one feels exhausted, all tend to deplete these hormones (indicated by the afflicted Sun in the horoscope).

When the Sun is afflicted in the horoscope, there is a lack of iodine and thus, a thyroid problem. A deficient thyroid may be involved in still birth, rheumatism, anemia, and diseases of the ear, nose and throat. It is known that the thyroid gland influences the metabolism of calcium, that is the way the body uses it and the amount it uses. Other illnesses involved when the Sun is afflicted in the horoscope can be found under the Vitamin and Mineral Therapeutic Applications on page 33.

The greatest value of exercise lies in its stimulating effect on the activity of the endocrine glands; perhaps, the thyroid in particular. When the endocrine glands are reduced in efficiency they contribute to the fatigue of old age (Sun afflicted and the person is not taking vitamin and mineral supplements to counteract it; thus the result is a deficiency).

Moon Afflicted...
Vitamins, Minerals

WHEN THE MOON is afflicted the body needs Vitamin B-2, B-6, Potassium, Germanium, and the proper salt-water balance.

Vitamin and Mineral Food Sources

Vitamin B-2: Whole grains, wheat germ, peanuts, lentils, watercress, cheddar cheese, mustard greens, milk, chicken, soybeans, green leafy vegetables, dandelion greens, turnip greens, cow's milk, buttermilk, salmon, fish, whole evaporated milk, organ meats (kidney, liver, lean beef heart and brains; veal, lamb, pork, calf), kale, almonds, eggs, dry navy beans, prunes, soy beans and lima beans.

Vitamin B-6: Green leafy vegetables, yeast, organ meats, bananas, whole grains.

Potassium: Cherries, potatoes, parsnips, turnips, apples, plums, bananas, red cabbage, eggplant, cucumbers, soybeans, grains, legumes, all green leafy vegetables, watercress, dnadelion, parsley, swiss chard, mustard greens, spinach, beet tops, tomatoes, endive, dill and watermelon.

Germanium: Garlic, ginseng, alfalfa and aloe vera.

Sodium: Avoid common table salt (sodium chloride) and use natural salt found in these foods: eggs, meat (lamb and calf liver), poultry (chicken, turkey), spinach, beets, celery, cucumbers, codfish, beef, milk, cream, butter, turnips, okra, potatoes, carrots, lettuce, cauliflower, cabbage, asparagus, broccoli, fresh peas, dry navy beans, fresh lima beans, wheat, barley, oats, rice, corn, beans in pod, huckleberries, gooseberries, strawberries, plums, peaches, oranges, lemons, cherries, bananas, apricots, apples, walnuts, unsalted peanuts, filberts, Brazil nuts, almonds, most breads, anchovies, and soy and tamari sauces.

Vitamin and Mineral Functions

Vitamin B-2: Necessary for fat, carbohydrate and protein metabolism, cell respiration, and formation of antibodies and red blood cells. Keeps the mucous lining of the digestive tract in healthy condition. Extremely important in eye health. Essential to the thymus gland and the production of the lymphatic cells.

Vitamin B-6: Necessary for fat, carbohydrate and protein metabolism, formation of antibodies, maintains sodium/potassium balance. It regulates the metabolism of the nervous system. It helps the bacterial flora which is beneficial to the proper development and good health of the teeth. Vitamin B-6 must be present in the digestive tract to digest and use properly the unsaturated fatty acids. If there is a shortage of these unsaturated fats (such as unhydrogenated vegetable oil) in the diet, lots of B-6 may be needed. Cholesterol is dissolved by the unsaturated fatty acids. If there are plenty of these fats in the diet, less Vitamin B-6 may be needed.

Potassium: Necessary for fluid balance. Controls activity of heart muscles, nervous system and kidneys. Necessary in construction of cells in body.

Germanium: It is an oxygen carrier and regulates the body's cellular oxygen levels, enhances the immune system, and restores the normal function of T cells and the numbers of antibody-forming cells. It is a trace mineral. It is not effective, if the blood is too acidic. It spares oxygen, and rids the body of toxic substances, i.e., mercury, lead, cadmium.

Sodium: Sodium is very solvent (dissolves easily). Chloride (the chemical content of table salt) serves no purpose in the body except that it may help form hydrochloric acid in the stomach, a certain amount of which is necessary for the digestion of proteins. The amount of salt necessary to produce hydrochloric acid in the stomach is amply supplied in food without any additional salt. Sodium regulates body fluid and acid base balance, and maintains nervous muscular, blood and lymph systems.

Vitamin and Mineral Deficiency Symptoms

Vitamin B-2: Eye problems, attacks in corners of mouth, digestive disturbances. The eyelids may smart and itch, the eyes may become tired and vision may be poor (cannot be improved by glasses). It may be difficult to see in dim light, along with a sensitivity to light (bright lights may bother the eyes). Fingernails break off easily. Nervous depression, loss of tissue tone, an unhealthy condition of the skin and perhaps one form of cataract.

Vitamin B-6: Nervousness, dermatitis, blood disorders, muscular weakness, insulin sensitivity, skin cracks, anemia, dandruff, hardening of the arteries, high blood pressure, and patchy, dull, dry skin.

Potassium: Poor reflexes, irregular heartbeat, dry skin, general weakness, poor circulation, constipation, and female problems.

Germanium: Tiredness. It should not be taken if ozone and other treatment of oxygen-giving supplements are used because it could strip the oxides and leave a toxic condition.

Sodium: An excess of salt in the diet can result in too much hydrochloric acid in the stomach which could produce stomach ulcers. It seems that, to a certain extent, sodium cancels out the excellent and necessary functions of calcium. Excess sodium chloride will enter into a struggle with calcium in the body and win. The result is less than an adequate amount of calcium for healthy teeth and bones. If large amounts of sodium chloride are taken, a good deal of it will be stored in the skin, mucous membranes and other tissues, and calcium will be liberated. Therefore, each sodium molecule retained in the tissues will diminish the calcium effect.

On the other hand, with a reduction of sodium chloride in the diet, the calcium action will prevail and lead up toward an anti-inflammatory effect. The secret of calcium lies in the relation of calcium taken with food to the other minerals, especially sodium, magnesium and phosphorus. If any of these is taken excessively, the calcium effect may be impaired. (I use Bone All supplements which have the necessary amount of minerals to blend with calcium.)

Sodium and potassium are natural enemies in the body's chemistry. A cell is in a state of repose when it rejects sodium and accepts potassium. It is in an active state when accepting sodium, which can affect the nerves and cause insomnia. Too much salt causes the body to lose potassium and the body needs potassium.

Excess sodium creates hardships for the kidneys, causes hypertension, high blood pressure, loss of hair, baldness, headaches and migraines. (There is a pressure on the nerves due to an increased flow of water to the tiny blood vessels of the head as a result of the water retention properties of sodium). Sodium creates a mineral imbalance when used to excess. Also, it may bring on sinus problems, infections, colds and other inflammations of the nasal passages. When the body is deficient in sodium, it causes muscle weakness and shrinkage, gas, nausea, and low blood pressure.

A high consumption of salt may be a predisposition to cancer.

Salt causes not only increased cramping of the capillaries, but it has been shown to be concentrated in body cells that are becoming increasingly cancerous, in reaction to which its biological opponent, potassium, fails.

Too much salt is involved in diseases of the kidney, liver, hardening of the arteries, stiff joints, diabetes, acidosis, kidney and gall stones, rheumatism, deafness, difficulty in childbirth and dropsy. (A disease which prompts the body to hoard water in abnormal amounts due to an excess amount of sodium; thus, a salt-free diet is needed).

Note: more than 8 grams a day of salt is injurious to the full utilization of proteins consumed. The kidneys cannot keep up with the job of eliminating this amount of salt and, as a result, it accumulates in the tissues; soon health problems develop.

Vitamin and Mineral Therapeutic Applications

Vitamin B-2: Cataracts, watering eyes, baldness, arthritis, emotional stress, indigestion.

Vitamin B-6: Atherosclerosis, high cholesterol, edema, palsy, Parkinson's disease, arthritis, cystitis, nervous disorders, obesity, emotional stress.

Potassium: High blood pressure, allergies, diabetes, diarrhea, colic in infants.

Germanium: It might help reduce tumors, good for arthritis.

Sodium: Good for low blood pressure. Everyone needs some natural salt in the system, or else the body's functioning would stop completely. It is necessary for the proper consistency of body fluids.

The Moon

The Moon has rulership over the fluidic (fluids) and lymphatic (lymph glands) systems of the body. The action of the back pituitary and thymus glands are influenced by the Moon. The alimentary tract's hormones, the medulla oblongata and the base of the brain (where magnetic energy is stored) are influenced by Moon aspects. The constitution is ruled by the Moon. The Moon governs the magnetic energy of the body. It has a strong influence over the eyes. When problems occur with the eyes, the Moon and Mars are both afflicted.

The back pituitary gland produces a secretion which causes contraction of all the arteries except those of the kidneys, and of the plain muscles of the bowels, the bladder, the womb and other organs. It has something to do with the metabolism of the carbohydrates. Its deficiency leads to obesity, and often is treated by the medical profession with injections of pituitrin and other hormones. A person who has an afflicted Moon in his horoscope (especially in the natal chart) usually has a weight problem due to the salt-water balance being off. A person who has an active (strong and harmonious Moon in the horoscope) back pituitary gland retains water less than the person who has a sluggish (afflicted Moon in the horoscope) back pituitary gland (this person craves lots of water and tends to retain it). The Moon rules the nutrient involved in the handling of water. Water is used in energy production but is more extensively used in the structure of the body which is more than half water.

The Moon also rules the hormones of the alimentary tract and the thymus gland. In nutrition the lymph cells take part in the absorption of fats by the intestines. When the Moon is afflicted in a horoscope, the back pituitary gland is overactive and causes water to be unduly retained. The thyroid needs to be stimulated to drive the water from the system. When the Moon is afflicted in an individual's chart, there is an accumulation of fluids. Petuitrin retains water. The salt-water balance is off and water is retained. Edema is involved where there is too much salt in the diet (it retains water in the tissues).

Mercury Afflicted...
Vitamins, Minerals

WHEN MERCURY IS afflicted the body needs Vitamin B-1, B-6, B-12, B-15, Choline, Niacin (no flush), Vitamin D-3, Calcium Citrate Supreme or Ultra Bone Up, Phosphorus, Potassium, Magnesium and Cell Food.

Note: Mineral oil prevents absorption of calcium. To assimilate calcium try boron, phosphorus, magnesium and Vitamin C (or eat or drink a citrus fruit 30 minutes before taking calcium. This markedly increases the ability of the body to absorb calcium). When a yeast problem exists, such as candida albicans, one cannot take brewer's yeast; therefore, a food source containing brewer's yeast is harmless in many, but not all cases.

Vitamin and Mineral Food Sources

Vitamin B-1, B-12, B-15, Niacin: Refer to the Sun, Page 23.

Vitamin B-6, Potassium: Refer to the Moon, page 37.

Choline (B Vitamin): Organ meats (kidney, liver, beef brains), snap beans, peanuts, lecithin, soy beans, fish, wheat germ, egg yolks, brewer's yeast.

Vitamin D: (The chief source of Vitamin D is sunlight which, falling on the bare skin, produces a substance which the body then changes into Vitamin D): Cod liver oil, irradiated oil, butter, cream, salmon, tuna, all fish liver oils, egg yolks, organ meats, fish, milk products, salad greens.

Calcium: Milk and dairy products, bone meal, clams, olives, tuna, yogurt, canned fish with bones (sardines, salmon), whole wheat, cheese, string beans, pecans, walnuts, oysters mustard greens, turnip tops, spinach, hazelnuts, broccoli, molasses, leeks, cabbage, parsnips, citrus fruits, all dark green vegetables, collard greens, dandelion greens, cottage cheese, celery, peas, okra, lima beans, lettuce, dates, soybeans, lemons, peanuts, brown rice, eggs, rye, raisins, dried prunes, almonds, kale, legumes, beans, dried figs, watercress, cauliflower, lentils, limes, and beet greens.

Phosphorus: Fish, meat, poultry, eggs, grains, legumes, prunes, baked potatoes, whole cereals, and cottage cheese.

Magnesium: Nuts, beans, green vegetables, whole grains, seed foods, seafood, cherries, figs, raisins, turnips, milk, legumes, spinach, whole cereals, natural brown or wild rice, soybeans, apples, plums, oranges, prunes, watercress, radishes, potatoes, barley, string beans, blackberries, blueberries, cabbage, celery, chinese cabbage, coconuts, dandelion greens, and oatmeal.

Vitamin and Mineral Functions

Vitamin B-1, B-12, B-15, Niacin: Refer to the Sun, pages 30, 31, 32.

Vitamin B-6, Potassium: Refer to the Moon, page 38.

Choline: It prevents the liver from becoming fatty. It contains a lipotropic substance which is attracted to fats and thus is useful in helping the body to manage them properly. Choline is powerful against the formation of cholesterol deposits. It is a vitamin necessary for fats to be transported to the body from the liver to the various fat deposits in the body. As a lipotropic agent it combines with fats or oils and thus hastens the removal of fat deposits. Because it protects the liver from harm, those who drink alcohol need choline in their systems. Choline aids memory and sharpens the mind. It helps prolong its effect on the blood sugar and prolongs the time before more insulin is needed. It plays a big part in the normal functioning of the pancreas.

Vitamin D: It is needed for the proper use of calcium and phosphorus by the body (it is necessary to assimilate calcium). It is for calcium and phosphorus metabolism (bone formation), heart action, and nervous system maintenance.

Calcium: For strong bones, teeth and muscle tissue; regulates heart beat, muscle action and nerve function, and blood clotting. Plenty of calcium in the diet prevents cramps and spasms, and it is good for preventing paralysis and epilepsy. It has been found to retard some cancerous tumors. It is necessary for the body to use Vitamin C correctly. Note: Caffeine, chocolate, and rhubarb rob the body of calcium.

Phosphorus: Bone development. Important in protein, fat, and carbohydrate utilization.

Magnesium: It is nature's laxative. Foods containing magnesium are especially beneficial to those who suffer from auto-intoxication and constipation as well as stiff and cracking joints. It gives the correct acid/alkaline balance needed by the body, and is important in the metabolism of carbohydrates, minerals, and sugar. Note: Caffeine, soft drinks and saturated fats rob the body of magnesium.

Vitamin and Mineral Deficiency Symptoms

Vitamin B-1, B-12: Refer to the Sun, pages 30, 31, 32.

Vitamin B-15, Niacin: Refer to the Sun, page 32.

Vitamin B-6, Potassium: Refer to the Moon, pages 37, 38.

Choline: Forgetful, absentminded (known to be lacking in patients with Alzheimer's disease), high bone pressure, bleeding stomach ulcers, liver and kidney problems, loss of memory. It is possible that a deficiency in Choline and Vitamin E produces muscular dystrophy. A lack of choline produces damage to the liver which interferes with the body's assimilation of Vitamin E. A choline deficiency calls for large doses of Vitamin E. (For Vitamin E, refer to Venus Afflicted, page 53.)

Vitamin D: A lack of Vitamin D prevents the proper use of lime and phosphorus from food, tends to affect the bones and teeth, (demineralization) and tends to promote faulty heart rhythm. Rickets, poor bone growth, nervous system affected, and irritability. It prevents clotting of the blood. In cases of osteoarthritis and osteoporosis a demineralization of the bones takes place. Its deficiency prevents the proper transmission of nerve impulses to the muscles.

Calcium: Soft, brittle bones, back and leg pains, tetany, heart palpitations, goiter, cataracts, spastic constipation, osteoporosis (Calcium that should appear in bones has disappeared, leaving the holes which bring on the osteoporosis.)

Diabetics usually lack calcium to such an extent that decalcification of the bones is common in elderly diabetics. Also, prolonged confinement in bed, or too much resting, depletes the calcium reserve. Calcium deficiency courts trouble as far as colds are concerned. A lack of calcium in the system affects the cilia. (This is the microscopic hair in the nose which covers the mucous membrane and moves back and fort like a field of wheat in the wind. They move the secretions of the nose into proper channels. The cilia need calcium for "backbone" to stand up to its job.)

Phosphorus: Poor bones and teeth, arthritis, rickets, appetite loss, and irregular breathing.

Magnesium: Nervousness, tremors, jitters, irritability, blood clots, easily aroused to anger, and loss of appetite.

Vitamin and Mineral Therapeutic Applications

Vitamin B-1, B-12, B-15, Niacin: Refer to the Sun, pages 30, 31, 32.

Vitamin B-6, Potassium: Refer to the Moon, page 38.

Choline: High blood pressure, hypoglycemia, Alzheimer's Disease, dizziness, headaches, ear noises, constipation, insomnia, liver and kidney problems, diabetes, atherosclerosis.

Vitamin D: Rickets, tooth decay, pyorrhea, colds, arthritis, osteomalacia, nearsightness, helps the parathyroid glands to function properly, prevents gall bladder trouble.

Calcium: Leg cramps, osteoporosis, arthritis, rheumatism, nervousness, menstrual cramps, back pains, spasms in the intestines, spastic colitis, spastic constipation, paralysis (polio, palsy, strokes), prevents, or helps epilepsy.

Phosphorus: Arthritis, stunted growth, stress, tooth and gum disorders.

Magnesium: Heart disease, alcoholism, high cholesterol, kidney stones, tooth decay, nervousness, depression.

Mercury

Mercury rules the mouth, tongue, brain, mucous membranes and the nervous system and currents. The action of the parathyroid glands and one hormone of the front pituitary gland is influenced by Mercury. The frequency of the electromagnetic vibrations of the body are handled by Mercury.

When Mercury is afflicted in the horoscope there are problems with the nerves, i.e., hypersensitivity, nervousness, shingles, insomnia. The calcium balance is disturbed which gives a great sensitiveness to the nerves and mucous membranes. The inability of the parathyroid glands to handle calcium in a major problem. The B family of vitamins help strengthen the parathyroid glands. Strains should be lessened on the nervous system. The vitality should be built up so that there will be more electromagnetic energy for the nerves.

When Mercury is discordant the nerves are unduly sensitive due to depletion of the supply of parathyrin. Mental activities, and especially mental strains and discords, affect the parathyroid glands, diminishing their secretion and permitting chemical imbalance chiefly due to improper assimilation of calcium. They also exhaust the nerve currents which, trying to meet the demands, become congested in certain areas due to the depletion of other areas.

The body does not preserve calcium as it does some other minerals. A brisk walk of several miles causes the body to store calcium. Walking, and other forms of exercise, promotes calcium metabolism. The body is quite wasteful of calcium. A considerable amount is excreted even when the body is not getting enough of it from food. There are large stores of calcium in the skeleton. When intake falls below the body's requirement, the bones suffer because calcium is withdrawn from the bones. Therefore, it is important to keep calcium intake high at all times because harm done by even a short period can result in damage that cannot be repaired. New bone matter is not formed in older people. However, calcium supplements appear to relieve pain and stop the progress of osteoporosis and other forms of bone loss. Make sure that the diet contains plenty of Vitamin C and D, phosphorus and calcium, thus preventing harmful calcium deposits to form in artery walls, or elsewhere in the body.

The lower the calcium intake, the greater the degree of gum disease. A high phosphorus and low calcium ratio can be part of a pyorrhea problem. Menopause and arthritic problems lie in the occurrence of an imbalance in the calcium-phosphorus ratio of the blood. Those who suffer with arthritis have diets which consist of high amounts of carbohydrates, low trace mineral intake and low consumption of foods rich in Vitamin B (also too many acid-forming foods - see pages 3 and 4). They eat refined and processed foods which contain elements which adversely affect the calcium-phosphorus ratio in the blood. Sugar is the surest way of knocking the calcium-phosphorus balance out of whack. It always boosts the calcium count while lowering the phosphorus; then, when the effect has worn off, the reverse occurs, and the phosphorus shoots up and the calcium is down; soon the individual is depressed. When Mercury is afflicted in the horoscope, calcium is beneficial to calm the jangled nerves.

Venus Afflicted...
Vitamins, Minerals

WHEN VENUS IS afflicted the body needs Vitamin E (if Iron is taken, they are incompatible, so Vitamin E and Iron need to be taken 12 hours apart), Iodine, Vitamin A (is toxic, therefore Carotene), Copper, Zinc, Niacin (no flush), Biotin, Inositol, Vital F (essential fatty acids), Vitamin K, and Octacosanol, Vitamin B-1, Leg Veins, Magnesium.

Note: When Venus is afflicted, do not eat sweets (sugar items) or carbohydrates because the body cannot assimilate them properly.

Vitamin and Mineral Food Sources

Iodine, Vitamin A: Refer to the Sun, pages 23, 24.

Niacin: Refer to the Sun, page 25.

Vitamin E: Butter, seed germ oil, seeds, milk, cheese, vegetable oils, green leafy vegetables, wheat germ, organ meats, eggs, legumes, brown rice, whole grains, cereal oils. Note: Vitamin E is destroyed in the presence of rancid fats (potato chips, salted nuts and many fried foods are dripping with rancid fat, especially those fried repeatedly). Chlorine destroys Vitamin E which is found in water. Many junk foods have been bleached with chlorine compounds.

Copper: Seafood (especially oysters), whole grains, green leafy vegetables, fresh calf's liver, almonds, pumpkin, string beans, potatoes, lettuce, asparagus, cabbage, cranberries, green peppers, tomatoes, kidney beans, wheat germ, peas, radishes, celery, cucumbers, lentils, corn, oats, barley, rye, molasses, asparagus, kale, grapes, beets, watercress.

Zinc: Eggs, whole grains, wheat germ, wheat bran, liver, legumes, poultry, dates, vegetables, dairy products, cheese, sunflower seeds, oysters, gelatin, apples, oranges, lemons, figs, grapes, chestnuts, pulpy fresh fruits, mineral water, honey, raspberries, loganberries, unblanched green vegetables, most sea fish, lean beef, milk, beets, bananas, celery, tomatoes, asparagus, carrots, radishes, potatoes, mushrooms, brewer's yeast, onions, brown rice, almonds, oatmeal, barley meal, rabbit, chicken, nuts, peas, beans, lentils, mussels, dried yeast.

Biotin (B vitamin): Yeast, organ meats, legumes, eggs, grain.

Inositol (B vitamin): Whole grains, citrus fruits, brewer's yeast, molasses, milk.

Vitamin F: Vegetable oils, wheat germ seeds, sunflower seeds, yeast, milk, fruits; corn sunflower, and safflower oils.

Vitamin K: Green leafy vegetables, milk, kelp, safflower oil, tomatoes, vegetable oils, alfalfa, spinach, oat sprouts, carrot tops, kale.

Octacosanol: Wheat germ oil.

Vitamin and Mineral Functions

Iodine, Vitamin A: Refer to the Sun, pages 23, 24.

Niacin: Refer to the Sun, page 25.

Vitamin E: It acts upon the glandular system, circulatory system, the proper development of the fetus, the blood vessels, the neuromuscular system, the locomotor and supporting systems, it also influences metabolism and, by its oxygen-giving and catalytic properties, protects the liver and mucous membranes of the stomach. It alleviates tiredness, increased working capacity and enhances mental efficiency.

Vitamin E is tied to the health of all muscles and it seems to have a part in increasing their oxygen supply; it is a muscle vitamin and plenty of Vitamin E is needed for muscle health. It treats various abnormalities of the muscles, red blood cells, liver and brain. It also treats diseases of the connective tissues.

Vitamin E protects fat soluble vitamins, helps prevent gall bladder troubles due to fatty foods, and relieves pain which is caused by a lack of oxygen in the heart, legs, feet, eyes, or any tissue where the circulation is decreased by fatty acids.

Vitamin E is effective in maintaining the health of the fetus, as well as in providing the fetus with the best possible atmosphere for normal development. It can be used as a means of preserving the fetus when threatened by miscarriage. It treats sterility and can help and cure menopause symptoms in women. It is good for dealing with disorders of the reproductive tract.

Cellular respiration is a Vitamin E function. It protects essential fatty acids, carotene (Vitamin A), the B vitamins, the pituitary gland, and sex hormone from being destroyed. Vitamin A is quickly used by oxygen if there is not enough Vitamin E. One of the functions of Vitamin E in the body is to bring about the synthesis of a substance called acetylcholine from choline and acetate. Vitamin E and B-5 are bound closely to choline in at least one body function.

Vitamin E decreases the body's need for oxygen. If some part of the body is in trouble because its oxygen supply is low, Vitamin E enables that particular part of the body to get along on less oxygen. The fact that Vitamin E can prolong the retention of oxygen in the blood stream is probably the key to its effectiveness in treating mental disorders. The brain needs an optimum supply of oxygen if it is to function properly. Perhaps, in some systems, the demands for oxygen elsewhere in the body exhaust the supply before the blood reaches the brain. This could be the result of an inadequate supply of oxygen in the first place, or because there is an inability to retain it in the blood long enough to meet all necessities.

Vitamin E is a substance normally circulating in the blood which prevents clots occurring inside the vessel. It helps improve the health of the circulatory system. It produces collateral circulation about the obstructed deep veins by calling into play the great unused networks of veins lying in wait for an emergency utilization. There are venous reserves and alpha tocopherol (found in Vitamin E) mobilizes them. Vitamin E produces new blood vessels around the site of an obstruction in a vessel so that the blood can continue to circulate there.

Vitamin E has the power of dilating the veins; that is, if they are narrowed by deposits so that the blood has trouble getting through, Vitamin E widens them. Vitamin E is an anti-thrombin, it has the power of retarding or preventing the coagulation of blood - a good guarantee against a clot in the brain or heart artery. Thus it can prevent death through thrombosis or a blood clot. It makes the tiny capillaries stronger so that hemorrhaging is unlikely. Thus the blood is kept in a normal state so that neither clots nor hemorrhages occur. It strengthens the heart and the blood vessel walls. It is probably the most important single item for preventing strokes. Because of its important oxygen-regulating function, Vitamin E has immediate and far-reaching effects on the entire heart and circulatory system. It improves tissue utilization of oxygen-conserving oxygen and helping tissues utilize available oxygen to best advantage becomes an important function of Vitamin E, especially when the daily oxygen supply gets exhausted with polluted air.

Vitamin E does not interfere with the normal clotting of blood in a wound and with the normal healing process. It actually accelerates the healing of burns and wounds. It is a natural oxygen-giving agent. Vitamin E prevents excessive scar tissue production. It is the key both to prevention and treatment of all those conditions in which a lack of blood supply due to thickened or blocked blood vessels or a lack of oxygen is a factor. It is used internationally in treatment of heart and other circulatory disorders.

Copper: Formation of red blood cells, bone growth; works with Vitamin C to form elastin.

Zinc: It is a trace mineral (barely traced in the body) and has been found to be an important part of the enzyme ``carbonic anhydrase.'' This enzyme takes an essential part in conveying carbon dioxide in the blood and is also concerned in some way with the body's acid-alkaline balance. All of these mechanisms would be considered hindered if the body lacked Zinc.

Zinc plays a bit part in the normal functioning of the pancreas. It helps prolong its effect on blood sugar; therefore zinc prolongs the time before more insulin is needed. Zinc is a must for sperm. In addition to the prostate gland, zinc is concentrated in the human body mostly in the liver and spleen, although the pancreas contains considerable amounts.

Biotin: It is directly involved in the assimilation of fat by the body. It must be present in the intestine in ample quantity or fat cannot be digested. Its function involves the formation of fatty acids, utilizing B vitamins, and helps utilize carbohydrate and protein metabolism.

Inositol: Vital for hair growth, lecithin formation, and fat and cholesterol metabolism. It s a powerful aid against the formation of cholesterol deposits - it lowers the cholesterol content of the blood.

Vitamin F: It functions in the respiration of body organs, resilience and lubrication of cells, blood coagulation, and glandular activity. Linolenic, linoleic and arachidonic acids are unsaturated fatty acids (Vitamin F). They have open links in their chain of atoms, and are ready, willing, and able to combine with other substances in the body. They can combine with other parts of food, help carry them through the blood vessels and are used in building cell structure. They can do all this because the open links in their chain of atoms invite other substances to join them in various chemical combinations. When oxygen is combined with the unsaturated fatty acids, an atom of oxygen moves into the empty link, joins itself chemically with the other atoms and the fat becomes rancid. Rancid fat in the diet destroys fat-soluble vitamins, whereas natural fats (i.e., sunflower seeds) carry with them oxygen-giving substances which prevent oxygen from turning the fat rancid.

Vitamin K: Important in formation of blood clotting agents, it is necessary for normal blood clotting and prevention of hemorrhaging. It is responsible for the proper coagulation of the blood. It helps prevent profuse bleeding. Bile must be present in the intestine or Vitamin K cannot be absorbed by the blood.

Octacosanol: It decreases blood cholesterol, assists in better muscle glycogen storage, improves endurance and reaction time, reduces high altitude stress and oxygen debt, and increases stability of basal metabolic rate under stress.

Vitamin and Mineral Deficiency Symptoms

Iodine, Vitamin A: Refer to the Sun, pages 28, 29.

Niacin: Refer to the Sun, page 32.

Vitamin E: Its lack in the mature female leads to a failure of the placental function and resorption of the fetus; in the adult male, its lack may lead to complete sterility, impotency, prostate trouble. During pregnancy and nursing, women suffering from a lack of Vitamin E are anemic, tired, somnolent, feel giddy, and are hardly able to accomplish mental or physical work.

Its deficiency symptoms are muscle wasting and abnormal deposits of fat in the muscles. It is possible that a lack of Vitamin E and choline could produce Muscular Dystrophy. A deficiency in choline produces damage to the liver which interferes with the body's assimilation of Vitamin E. When there is a choline deficiency, a large doses of Vitamin E is needed. Note: Those who should not use large doses of Vitamin E are hyperthyroid patients, and those who suffer from rheumatic heart and high blood pressure. Always check with a doctor first.

Its lack causes gastrointestinal disease and heart disease, and it could be involved in osteoarthritis. The osteoarthritis is brought about by an impaired mechanism that upsets the normal balance inside the body cell. It starts with a deficiency of oxygen in the cell and then goes on to destroy the cell.

Copper: General weakness, skin sores, and impaired respiration.

Zinc: Retarded growth, prolonged wound healing, delayed sexual maturity, diabetes, decrease in hair growth, seriously affects reproduction and can cause a lack of sperm, prostate trouble. It is possible that if there is insufficient zinc that the body cannot properly absorb the B vitamins which can also lead to a deficiency in the B vitamins as well as Zinc.

Biotin: Dry, grayish skin, depression, muscle pain, fatigue and poor appetite. Caffeine creates a deficiency.

Inositol: High cholesterol, hair loss, skin problems, constipation, eye abnormalities, caffeine creates a deficiency.

Vitamin F: Brittle nails and hair, dandruff, diarrhea, varicose veins, underweight, gallstones, acne and prostate trouble.

Vitamin K: Tendency to hemorrhage, gum disease; aspirin and other drugs containing salicylic acid block the action of Vitamin K in the body. Vitamin K is directly affected by anything that goes wrong with the gall bladder.

Octacosanol: Fatigue.

Vitamin and Mineral Therapeutic Applications

Iodine, Vitamin A, Niacin: Refer to the Sun, pages 33, 34.

Vitamin E: It can help with hot flashes, painful, or irregular menstruation. Alpha tocopherol (found in Vitamin E) has been shown to be an oxygen-conserving agent. This alone would make it valuable in pregnancy. The placenta can also be regarded as a sponge, a net of capillaries, their being kept intact is vital to the life of the fetus. Vitamin E is beneficial for the menopause, female problems, and prevents reproductive disorders. The natural hormones which occur in wheat germ oil are partly responsible for its good effect.

Vitamin E may reduce the need for Digitalis for the heart and, in cases of thrombosis, the taking of Vitamin E can save lives by preventing blood from forming clots. It helps prevent cardiovascular disease and reduces blood clots, helps heart disease, angina, arteriosclerosis, atherosclerosis and Buerger's disease. (A disease of the blood vessels in which the inner linings of both arteries and veins become inflamed. There is also clogging of the blood due to blood clots. The disease affects the legs and feet, in general.)

Vitamin E has been known to work favorably against muscle-wasting in leprosy. It aids those with epilepsy mental disorders, diabetes (it may reduce the need for insulin), cataracts (also need Vitamin B), peptic ulcer, varicose veins, intracranial birth damage, enlarged prostate, burns, scars, headaches, hypertension, gangrene, phlebitis and dermatological problems. It is useful in opthalmology, myopia (near-sightedness—a disease of the connective tissue for which, along with the amino acids and a high protein diet, Vitamin E has been an aid), and has been known to help Mongoloid children (along with other vitamins). Also those with cystic fibrosis, who have low levels of Vitamin E in the blood, have been given high levels of E and have been helped (along with other vitamins). Vitamin E has helped those with poor circulation and in polio patients relieves numbness, tingling and cramps in the extremities.

Copper: Anemia, baldness, edema.

Zinc: Helps eliminate cholesterol deposits, atherosclerosis, hypoglycemia, diabetes, infertility, internal, and external wounds.

Biotin: Baldness, leg cramps, dermatitis and exzema.

Inositol: Atherosclerosis, high cholesterol, baldness, obesity. It gives a better absorption of foods and causes a marked increase in the intestinal movements, thus is good for constipation.

Vitamin F: Leg ulcers, eczema, psoriasis, asthma, rheumatoid arthritis, heart disease and softens cholesterol.

Vitamin K: Menstrual problems, gallstones, hemorrhages; promotes the clotting of blood and helps prevent profuse bleeding. (This benefits those with hemophilia, pre-menstrual syndrome and chronic bleeders.)

Octacosanol: Improves oxygen utilization, lowers blood cholesterol, and may be helpful for those who experience muscle pain after exercise and have poor exercise or lowered tolerance.

Venus

Venus rules the venous blood and the veins, skin and hair. It also has a decided influence over the pharyngeal tonsil, sex organs, ovaries, thyroid, the female gonad glands, and upper kidneys. Also Venus rules the energy-yielding carbohydrates which embrace the sugars and starches. They are the most economic energy foods and are stored in small amounts as glycogen, or animal starch, and for more adequate storage are transformed into fat. Those who have an afflicted Venus in their horoscopes have difficulty in assimilating sugars and starches, and could attract hypoglycemia or diabetes.

When Venus is afflicted there are irritants in the blood stream and the walls of the veins are weakened. The chemical imbalance is due to imperfect functioning of the thyroid and gonad glands (the action of these glands is influenced by Venus). The diet should be such as to alkalize the blood stream and free it from irritants such as acids. Emotional stress should be avoided, and a poised attitude cultivated. Otherwise, thyroxine is poured into the blood stream and this stimulates the heart and contracts the blood vessels. The hormone of the gonad glands does likewise through its action upon adrenalin. Thus, Vitamin E helps prevent these problems from arising.

When Venus is discordant, a person is hypersensitive; thus the skin and hair are affected. The secretion of the thyroid gland is directly involved in all skin problems. The body needs Vitamin E and sufficient copper (and the other vitamins listed) for blood building. When Venus is afflicted the kidneys may be affected; they are chiefly responsible for filtering toxins and acids from the blood stream and when there is a disturbance which prevents the proper filtering and handling of the urine, health problems manifest. Thyroxin tends to drive water from the body.

When Venus is discordant it is also important to be careful to avoid contracting social diseases (syphilis; also Mars, Saturn afflicted), Gonorrhea (also Mars, Neptune afflicted), herpes, AIDS (also Mars, Saturn, Neptune and Pluto afflicted). When a person has AIDS the venous blood is affected and the body needs plenty of the vitamins listed for Venus afflictions, especially Vitamin E and all the other oxygen-giving vitamins and supplements.

Mars Afflicted...
Vitamins, Minerals

WHEN MARS IS afflicted the body needs Vitamin A (Carotene), B-1, B-2, B-6, B-12 (or Cracked Cell Chlorella, if the body cannot tolerate B-12), Folic Acid (B-9), Niacin (no flush), Vitamin C (rose hips), Vitamin E, K, P (Bioflavonoids), Iron (take Vitamin E and Iron 12 hours apart), Zinc, Copper, Manganese, Pancreatin (quadruple strength), Betaine Hydrochloric Acid, L. Carnitine (an amino acid), L. Arginine (an amino acid), Sod-3, Potassium, grapefruit seed extract, Bladder Care (for the bladder), Kidney Care (for the kidneys), and/or Malic Acid (for the muscles).

Note: When Mars is afflicted, care should be taken with protein foods—less intake but variety because there is difficulty handling protein, which is not digested. Pancreatin helps alleviate this problem. Hydrochloric Acid aids digestion, especially for people over age 40. With a discordant Mars, there may be less energy; therefore, "Bee Pollen" could help perk up the energy, or Cell Food, Cracked Cell Chlorella (easy to digest, oxygen-giving, a wonderful source of energy, a healing agent, and good for the immune system). Consult a physician before taking Vitamin K and Copper.

Vitamin and Mineral Food Sources

Manganese, Vitamin A: Refer to the Sun, page 24.

Vitamin B-1, B-12, Folic Acid, Niacin: Refer to the Sun, pages 24, 25.

Vitamin B-2, B-6: Refer to the Moon, page 37.

Vitamin E, Copper, Zinc: Refer to Venus, pages 51, 52.

Vitamin K, Octacosanol: Refer to Venus, page 52.

PABA (Para-amini-Benzoiac-Acid, and a B Vitamin): Liver, yeast, molasses, wheat germ.

Vitamin C: Grapefruit, oranges, lemons, limes, apples, peaches, raspberries, blueberries, strawberries, apricots, bananas, tomatoes, kale, soybeans, beef, calf and lamb liver, asparagus, radishes, turnips and their tops, pineapple, white rutabagas, mangos, papaya, persimmons, tangerines, blackberries, gooseberries, black and white grapes, black currants, prunes, radishes, kohlrabi, spinach, watercress, mustard greens, rose hip products, broccoli, brussels sprouts, raw cabbage, dandelion greens, red cayenne pepper, beet greens, melon, cantaloupe, cauliflower, red and green peppers, parsley, summer squash and potatoes. Note: Cabbage and other foods contain trace amounts of cyanide but also contain large amounts of Vitamin C (the warrior against cyanides).

Vitamin C is highly perishable and disappears rapidly from foods, especially when they wilt or rot, or are washed away completely when soaked in water before cooking or eating. (Vitamin C is sensitive to heat).

Vitamin P (Bioflavonoids): Paprika, apricots, blackberries, cherries, black currants, summer squash, black and white grapes, lemon, orange, grapefruit, parsley, prunes, plums, buckwheat and rose hip products.

Iron: Meats (lean beef), organ meats (liver), fish, green leafy vegetables, milk, avocados, oatmeal, barley, rye, molasses, eggs, beans, dried lentils, turnip tops, red and white cabbage, spinach, beets, lettuce, raw carrots, cherries, currants, blackberries, strawberries, loganberries, onions, oysters, corn, beet greens, all nuts (especially English walnuts, almonds), celery, watercress, dried beans, peas, and prunes, whole wheat, oats, parsley, dandelion greens (more iron than spinach) and all greens.

Pancreatin: Tablet form.

Beta-Pepsin: Betaine Hydrochloric Acid with Pepsin (capsule or tablet form).

Protein: Meat, fish, eggs, poultry, dairy products, milk, cheese, lentils, beans, cereals, buckwheat, whole grains, peas, soybeans, quinoa, amaranth and whole wheat. Note: Protein from vegetables, fruits, nuts, seeds, beans, and some wheat products do not contain all of the essential amino acids; however, soybeans and the seed or pasta form of Quinoa are complete proteins with all of the essential amino acids. Replace pasta made from white flour with amaranth or quinoa (sold at health food stores).

Amino Acids: These foods are the richest in protein. There are 22 essential amino acids but these are the most important:

Glutamic Acid and Glycine: Brewer's yeast, milk, casein (milk protein), eggs, lean beef, lamb, veal, chicken, haddock, fish, liver (beef, calves, chicken), Kidney beans, lentils, peanuts, soybeans, filberts, cottonseed flour and meal, corn, and whole wheat flour.

Alanine: In all of the preceding except eggs, chicken, haddock, fish and filberts.

Carnitine: An amino acid found highest in muscle and organ meat.

SOD (Super-Oxide-Dismutase): Kale, spinach, dandelion greens, collard greens, broccoli, comfrey, wheat sprouts.

Vitamin and Mineral Functions

Manganese, Vitamin A, B-1: Refer to the Sun, page 24.

Vitamin B-12, Folic Acid, Niacin: Refer to the Sun, pages 24, 25.

Vitamin B-2, B-6: Refer to the Moon, page 37.

Vitamin E: Refer to Venus, pages 53, 54, 55.

Copper, Zinc, Octacosanol, Vitamin K: Refer to Venus, pages 55, 56, 57.

PABA: Protein metabolism, red blood cell formation,healthy intestines, hair coloring, sunscreen.

Vitamin C: The main and most important function of Vitamin C is that it assists in the formation of collagen generally for the maintenance of integrity and stability of the connective tissues, including bones, cartilage, muscle and vascular tissue. Collagen is protein made exclusively of amino acids; it is the substance that is important in all connective tissue, it is the material that makes gelatin when bone and cartilage is boiled. It is widely distributed throughout most tissues and is found in large amounts in bone, cartilage, tendons and skin. Collagen depends for its formation on a sufficiency of Vitamin C. It is necessary to have plenty of protein in the diet (because it is made of protein) to prevent damage to the collagen (the substance that holds cells together). Vitamin C must be present to form the cement that holds these cells together. The intercellular material is kept in repair by Vitamin C. When there is not enough Vitamin C, cell material flakes off and forms a kind of garbage which has no place to go. The intercellular cement will disintegrate gradually and the cells will fall apart.

Vitamin C is necessary for the normal mineralization of bone and teeth and, especially the formation of bone tissue. It is important to the prevention of osteoporosis (porous bone in which the spaces between deposits of mineral have become so large that the bone looks honeycombed. It is bone that is decalcified because calcium has been lost from them, thus, the bone is soft and easily liable to fracture).

Vitamin C contributes to the health of the blood vessels in two ways: 1)By its ability to build up the actual blood vessel tissues so they are strong and flexible; then maintenance by preserving the strength of the capillary walls so they will be in good condition. 2)Its ability to decrease collections of cholesterol. Vitamin C alone is necessary to prevent fatty degeneration of the liver. Ample quantities of Vitamin C cause the harmful deposits of fat to disappear rapidly.

Vitamin C is important in the sound and rapid healing of wounds, the prevention of hemorrhaging, and the building of a barrier against germ invasion. It contributes to building up disease fighters or antibodies in the blood stream and neutralizes toxins in the blood; it helps to build a natural immunity to infectious diseases and poisons. Vitamin C does its work in the white blood corpuscles which the body calls out to fight infection. In cases of fever, or hard physical exertion, the body uses up Vitamin C much faster than usual. Vitamin C gives the body a chance to knock out infection by destroying the toxins in the blood stream that can be damaging to nerve tissue. Thus the poisons taken in every day through food and atmosphere are neutralized. In the process of fighting germs and poisons, Vitamin C is destroyed (oxidized, burned, and used up in the battle) immediately in the performance of its task; therefore, it must be constantly replenished. Any excess of Vitamin C is carried away by the kidneys.

The presence of Vitamin C is of utmost importance in the entire oxidation process that takes place in the cells. By threefold, Vitamin C increases the oxidation-enzymes in the blood, which are so important to the whole oxidation process. Vitamin C is concentrated in many tissues of the body, such as the adrenal glands. It is needed to keep the mucous lining of the digestive tract in good condition.

Vitamin C is not stored in the body; it could be used up hourly, depending upon lifestyle—the amount of poison that enters the body daily. Smokers need Vitamin C often. Vitamin C cannot function well in the absence of Vitamin P (Bioflavonoids); therefore, it is best to take it at the same time.

Vitamin P (Bioflavonoids): It appears to affect the capillary system directly, perhaps participating as a principal in the ``wear and tear" of a part or all of the capillary system, inhibiting its degeneration and taking part in its regeneration, specifically as far as the intercellular cement (the substance between the body cells which holds them together) is concerned. Vitamin P strengthens capillaries and keeps connective tissue of cells healthy and helps to maintain capillary and cell wall permeability. It is beneficial in treating capillary injuries of all kinds, especially bruising. It has been proven to be effective after cosmetic surgery if the individual takes about 12,000 units a day for two weeks before; after surgery there will be no, or very few, black and blue marks on the skin. It is used to treat certain conditions involving hemorrhaging inside the skin. It helps prevent the possibility of a stroke. It helps the body utilize Vitamin C. It does not take part in body processes without Vitamin C being present. Vitamin C and P seem to be closely related to the health of the blood vessels; they prevent hemorrhages by keeping the walls of the blood strong and healthy; they have the capacity to correct abnormal capillary fragility and permeability; they are supposedly good for hemorrhage in the retina of the eye, and cerebral or brain hemorrhages. Together they keep the body from bruising easily, bring down high blood pressure and diminish fatigue.

Iron: Organic iron removes waste products and assists greatly in cleansing the blood stream. It is good for hemoglobin formation, improves blood quality, increases resistance to stress and disease and gives energy. Note: Inorganic Iron should never be taken as it is an irritant to the kidneys.

Pancreatin: Aids the body in the digestion of protein.

Beta-Pepsin: It gives the necessary hydrochloric acid needed in the stomach to digest Vitamin A.

Protein: Involved in the formation of bone. It is necessary for the muscles and walls to function properly. Essential for the growth and repair of tissue. Gives physical energy when digested properly.

Carnitine: Utilized as a material which transfers fatty acids across the membranes of the mitochondria (the ``lungs" of the cell) where they can be used as a source of fuel to generate energy. An important regulatory effect upon fat metabolism in heart and skeletal muscles.

SOD: A protein and enzyme that is in all body cells and fights the harmful free radicals in the body. It takes these radicals and by deactivation turns them (along with nature's catalase) into stable oxygen and hydrogen peroxide, and then into water and oxygen. Note: Catalase without sod and sod without catalase is toxic.

Vitamin and Mineral Deficiency Symptoms

Manganese, Vitamin A: Refer to the Sun, pages 28, 29.

Vitamin B-1, B-12: Refer to the Sun, pages 30, 31, 32.

Folic Acid, Niacin: Refer to the Sun, page 32.

Vitamin B-2, B-6: Refer to the Moon, page 39.

Vitamin E, Copper, Zinc: Refer to Venus, pages 56, 57.

Vitamin K, Octacosanol: Refer to Venus, page 57.

PABA: Digestive disorders, fatigue, depression, nervousness, irritability, constipation, and gray hair.

Vitamin C: A deficiency destroys the body's ability to rebuild tissues and fibers such as the tissues of the gums. It tends to prevent the proper formation and maintenance of teeth and tends toward bleeding of the mouth and gums by making the capillaries so fragile that they bleed easily, i.e., pyorrhea, periodontal disease and tartar (placque) on the teeth Lack of Vitamin C leads to a breakdown of body tissues. The teeth become loose in cases of scurvy (a Vitamin C deficiency disease) because the cementing substance holding them in has liquefied (there is not enough Vitamin C to keep the cementing substance in good repair).

In a Vitamin C deficiency, instability and fragility of all tissues is believed to be caused by the breakdown of intercellular cement substance, resulting in easy rupture of any kind and all of the connective tissues (including the discs of the backbone, ligaments, small sacs in the interior of the joints and the cartilage which helps in the movement of the joints). If Vitamin C is lacking, this intercellular cement will disintegrate gradually and the cells will fall apart. When there is inadequate formation of the intercellular material, or collagen, the cells remain immature and blood vessels do not easily penetrate the poorly developed granulation tissue. When the cement of the cells is missing, tissues tend to give way. Skin breaks develop, and capillaries and veins rupture under the stress of their normal job; stomach linings become weak enough to be attacked by gastric juices, and the result is ulcers. A lack of Vitamin C delays the healing of ulcers.

A Vitamin C deficiency produces a fatty liver. Because Vitamin C has lipotropic properties it can help the fatty liver. In cases of polio the strength of the capillary walls is found to be diminished. The infection which is more safely contained in them tends to "leak" through the walls, attacking the more susceptible nerve cells.

When Vitamin C is deficient in the diet, certain skeletal tissues form a fluid material rather than dentine and bone (their natural products). If Vitamin C is given, this material rapidly gels or solidifies. Lack of Vitamin C causes the skeletal tissue cells to become useless. This results in less oxygen consumption by the cells, reduced digestive juices in the stomach, reduced content of hormones in the adrenal glands, retarded formation of blood and decreased ability to fight infection.

When there is a lack of oxygen, the body does not assimilate Vitamin C properly and there is a collagen breakdown. A lack of oxygen is why body organs grow old, permitting arteries and veins to harden, and causing strokes and degeneration of the brain. Thus aging goes hand in hand with a Vitamin C deficiency.

When there is not enough Vitamin C in the urinary tracts, mucous lining scales off and forms the nucleus of stones (kidney, gall bladder, and those in other parts of the body - even the calcium deposits that bring hardening of the arteries and arthritis). An injection of insulin lowers the level of Vitamin C in the blood and seems to redistribute it to other parts of the body. A vitamin C deficiency is involved in leukemia, tuberculosis, "conduction deafness," cataract (there is little or no Vitamin C in the lens of the eye), infection, slow healing wounds, bruising, aching joints, nose bleeds, and poor digestion. Also, cancer may develop if there is a lack of Vitamin C (those with cancer have been found to lack Vitamin C in their body).

The more sprays, chemicals, insecticides and other poisons the body is subjected to, the more Vitamin C is needed to stay healthy. Vitamin C in the body is destroyed the instant these poisons come into contact with it. The toxic fumes of tobacco also destroy or neutralize to a large extent what little Vitamin C is taken in the food. The smoking of one cigarette, as ordinarily inhaled, tends to neutralize in the body about 25 milligrams of Vitamin C or the Vitamin C content of one orange. The caffeine in coffee, soft drinks, chocolate, etc., destroys Vitamin C.

To avoid a Vitamin C deficiency take extra Vitamin C if feeling jittery or angry or things are not going smoothly; bosses, superiors or loved ones have been too demanding; temperature is too hot or too cold; fitful sleep; cuts or burns; alcohol or tobacco has been used or foods eaten that contained chemical additives or preservatives; improper ventilation in a room, or breathed fumes from a car, aerosol spray can or cleaning fluid; or if the body suffers from any joint disease, is pregnant or scheduled for surgery; or shocks, upsets, emotional turmoils, upheavals, a crisis or any drastic event is experienced.

Vitamin P (Bioflavonoids): Similar to Vitamin C, easy bruising, and bleeding. When Vitamin P is discontinued, the capillary fragility increases.

Iron: Anemia (pale skin, fatigue), constipation, and breathing difficulties.

Pancreatin: If protein is not digested, fatigue may be a problem and illnesses may be attracted. The disease cancer is, partially, a protein metabolism problem.

Beta-Pepsin: Its deficiency could lead to ulcers or stomach problems.

Protein: Problems with the bone, muscles, tissue repair. You are tired all of the time, and seem to have no physical strength when there is a protein deficiency. When there is not enough protein in the diet, the muscles of the walls of the stomach and intestines cannot function, and the flabbiness which results may cause the entire intestinal structure to "fall" so that organs are displaced and constipation results. Foods remain undigested when the flabby walls of the intestine cannot contract normally. The blood vessels are made of protein, as are other parts of the body, and if enough protein is not available in the diet to keep them from being flabby they will gradually waste away just as muscles do. Edema is one of the most important symptoms of protein deficiency.

Carnitine: In the absence of proper carnitine levels within the cell, the fatty acids are poorly metabolized and can build up within the cell of the surrounding medium, thereby leading to elevated blood fat and triglyceride levels, infiltration of the liver with fat, depressed muscle carnitine levels with generalized spleen and liver enlargement, and muscle wasting. A deficiency can lead to increased risk to small vessel disease, kidney problems and the inability to walk without pain.

The spermatozoa from lysine depletion might make a person infertile. Adequate levels of carnitine are necessary for energy metabolism within the sperm for proper motility and fertility. Note: Vitamin C is needed with Carnitine.

SOD: When harmful free radicals are left unchecked, they attach to supporting tissue collagen. Thus tissues become stiff, skin wrinkles, and it causes deposits to form on the arterial walls. Sod could delay a major cause of aging.

Vitamin and Mineral Therapeutic Applications

Manganese, Vitamin A, B-1, B-12, Folic Acid, Niacin: Refer to the Sun, pages 33, 34.

Vitamin B-2, B-6: Refer to the Moon, page 39.

Vitamin E, Copper, Zinc, Vitamin K, Octacosanol: Refer to Venus, pages 58, 59.

PABA: Baldness, burns, gray hair, dry skin, sunburn, burns, wrinkles, vitiligo (a disease in which smooth white patches form on various parts of the body due to loss of natural pigment).

Vitamin C: If there is plenty of Vitamin C in the diet, there is far less chance that whatever the fat eaten is going to collect in the liver to do deadly damage there. If the liver has been damaged, Vitamin C will immediately cause it to begin to reconstruct those cells once again. Vitamin C aids high cholesterol.

Vitamin C increases the strength of the capillaries, thus is helpful in polio. It is good for the nerves, teeth, gums, bones and eyes. In fact, bleeding bums may return to normal. And in matters of the eyes, there are large amounts of Vitamin C in the lenses and other parts of the normal and healthy eye.

Vitamin C is used in treatment for various contagious and infectious diseases, and is beneficial for infections in general. Allergies, wounds, and stress have all been helped by Vitamin C.

It helps abort colds, aids in heart disease, has helped those with undulant fever (Brucellosis), atherosclerosis, arthritis, acne, high blood pressure, tuberculosis, pneumonia, diphtheria, rheumatic fever, whooping cough, and resistance to infection. Large doses have brought back hearing to many people.

Vitamin P (Bioflavonoids): It may reduce pressure, e.g., on the eyeball in glaucoma or bruising (after surgery or when injured). It preserves the state of the blood vessels, preventing strokes and high blood pressure. It helps alleviate stress. Vitamin P can be used effectively in treating abnormal capillary fragility and bleeding. It helps bleeding gums, ulcers, hemorrhoids, rheumatism, arthritis, bursitis, and along with Vitamin C is a powerful agent against the common cold, flue, and asthma.

Vitamin P may be helpful in reducing cancer growths. It may be used in the treatment of cases involving hemorrhaging due to disease, drugs which the patient was taking for the disease or poisoning. Labyrinthitis (a disease of the inner ear, characterized by varying degrees of dizziness, loss of balance and nausea) can be helped by Vitamin P in cases where something goes wrong with the capillaries in the ear.

Iron: Anemia, colitis, menstrual problems.

Pancreatin: Has helped in cancer.

Beta-Pepsin: Helps stomach and ulcer problems.

Protein: When digested properly and not deficient in the diet, it has helped edema, builds strong muscles (gives good muscle coordination), aids physical energy (strength improved) and aids the formation of bone.

Carnitine: It is an agent to improve fat metabolism and to reduce blood triglycerides. Neuromuscular diseases (Muscular Dystrophy and so forth) have been aided by it. Helpful to those people who want to improve fatty acid metabolism due to metabolic obesity problem.

SOD: Good for energy, arthritis and the heart (could restore damaged tissues after a heart attack), it deactivates radiation effects and could be a preventive against aging.

Mars

The gonad glands are influenced by Mars. The muscles (muscular system) and the red corpuscles of the blood are ruled by Mars. It governs the adrenal glands: Mars is involved in the secretion of both adrenalin and cortin by the adrenal glands. As these are the chief chemicals with which the body fights toxic conditions and invasions by bacteria, an afflicted Mars in the horoscope predisposes to surgical operations, accidents, blood poison, fevers (hot and dry feverish complaints, such as AIDS victims have), cysts, boils inflammations, wounds, abrasions, cuts and tears, and tends to acute and painful diseases. Also abscesses and various types of infection. The affection occurs because the body does not have at hand the chemicals with which it otherwise would oust the invaders. Fever is the result of adrenalin and cortin trying to rid the body of the enemy agent and neutralize its toxins. When you have a cold, the blood stream is unable to oust the invading organisms. A bacterial infection is a toxic condition usually involving temporary irritation, excitement or a spurt of exertion which releases adrenalin. Emotional upsets of any kind affect the chemical balance of the blood stream. When Mars is afflicted and when these two chemicals are exhausted (depleted), toxins remain unneutralized in the blood stream and infection, attracted by a discordant Mars, easily gains a foothold and inflammation develops. (The disease AIDS is an example - Mars afflicted is always involved in the disease AIDS). Note: The ability of the blood to coagulate is largely determined by the amount of adrenalin present in the blood stream.

Note: Mars rules sex. When Mars is afflicted, social diseases e.g., AIDS can be easily attracted if a person is involved in a sexual relationship.

Mars rules the muscle building proteins. Proteins, such as

those obtained from egg whites, curds of milk, lean meat, gluten of wheat, legumes and so forth, are chiefly used to build or repair tissue. They are also used in the manufacture of the various enzymes which act as catalysts. And, although expensive fuels, some are used for this purpose commonly, and when the other fuels are lacking the lean tissues of the body are thus employed. When Mars is afflicted there is difficulty in digesting (handling) protein; it is a metabolism problem. The low output of cortin hormone results in the incomplete metabolism of protein foods, with an accumulation of toxins. One needs a variety of proteins that can be used in building new red blood cells to replace those destroyed (especially, when Mars is discordant in the horoscope). The adrenal glands should be favored as much as possible by avoiding strain or excitement; then they can supply additional adrenalin and cortin. The kidneys are chiefly responsible for filtering toxins and acids from the blood stream. Too much protein places a strain both on the kidneys and the cortin supply. Alcohol (ruled by Mars) is very hard on the kidneys.

Mars rules the bile and gall bladder. When the blood stream is acid it may cause inflammation of the bile ducts and the gall bladder. Then, it is necessary to alkalize the blood stream. A diet rich in alkaline-forming elements is helpful. An acid blood stream causes the blood vessels to contract, and thus raises the blood pressure. When Mars is afflicted, the adrenalin, and cortin supply is depleted and an acid or toxic condition develops. Uric acid can develop in the blood from the nuclei of meat (ruled by Mars) and thus a chemical imbalance is present in which the adrenalin and cortin supply are insufficient to neutralize the acidity of the blood stream. Excess meat consumption is bad and all acid producing foods should be avoided (refer to page 3 and 4).

When Mars is afflicted in the horoscope, there is an imbalance which may affect the male gonad glands, such as in AIDS. The hormone of the gonad gland stimulates the heart and contracts the blood vessels through its action upon adrenalin. Cortin and adrenalin contract the arterial blood vessels, stimulate the circulation and raise the blood pressure (ruled by Mars) even more violently than does thyroxine. The feeling of anger, irritation, haste, strain, hurry, pressure, demands, mental stress, or physical exhaustion (the forcing of oneself to continue after one feels exhausted), releases adrenalin and withdraws the blood from the digestive tract (stomach). Thus, do not eat when the emotions are aroused to any of these states or if your mind is over active. A mental state free from excitement, fear, and temperamental outbursts, or any other emotion or strain is a must; otherwise, these emotional upsets cause the body to release and use up its adrenalin and cortin supply. Note: A strong and afflicted Mars tends to cause high blood pressure and those who have it are the excitable type just described.

Mars Afflicted...Vitamins, Minerals

Jupiter Afflicted...
Vitamins, Minerals

WHEN JUPITER IS afflicted the body needs Vitamin B-2, B-5, B-6, B-12, B-15, Biotin, Choline, Inositol, Niacin (no flush), Vitamin E, Vitamin F (essential fatty acids), Magnesium, Liver Care (detoxes the liver), Red Yeast Rice capsules (to reduce cholesterol)), Kyolic garlic (to reduce cholesterol and for caradio-vascular, purifies the blood stream), Lecithin, L. Phenylalaline (to reduce weight), Chromium Picolinate (to reduce weight), L. Carnitine (to reduce weight), Sulphur (cnsult a physician before taking), Artichoke Extract (for the liver and gall bladder), and to reduce tumors (Essiac, Cell Forte with IP 6, Graviola Gamma bama, Sour Sop).

Note: When Jupiter is afflicted, Evening Primrose Oil is beneficial. It is a natural source of Gamma Linolenic Acid and of Linoleic Acid, polyunsaturated fatty acids necessary to components of all body cells and for the production of beneficial prostaglandins (the chemical regulator of many body functions) in the body. Modern diet and lifestyles may reduce efficiency of the conversion of essential fatty acids into Gamma-Linoleic

Acid (GLA). GLA is directly converted to prostaglandin. It is beneficial for losing weight, getting fat out of the body and for the heart and so forth. For those who have Jupiter afflicted, it is best to take a water soluble Vitamin E. Consult a physician before taking Sulphur.

Vitamin B-17 (Laetrile, Amygdalin) has been reported to decrease and/or destroy tumors, especially cancerous ones. However, it may be difficult to purchase. Its food sources are almonds, raspberry jam, apricots, apples, lima beans, buckwheat and wheat grass.

Thiotic Acid (Thiox) can oxidize serious poisons such as Mercury toxemia, and destroying angel mushroom poisoning. It helps metabolize liver toxins, chemical hypersensitivity syndrome, heavy metal toxicity, diabetic neuropathy, chronic aggressive hepatitis, elevated liver enzymes, other chronic liver diseases, alcoholism, and narcotic addictions as well as various poisonings.

Vitamin and Mineral Food Sources

Vitamin B-5, B-12, B-15, Niacin, Co-enzyme Q-10: Refer to the Sun, pages 24, 25.

Vitamin B-2, B-6: Refer to the Moon, page 37.

Choline, Magnesium: Refer to Mercury, pages 43, 44.

Vitamin E, Zinc: Refer to Venus, pages 51, 52.

Biotin, Inositol, Vitamin F, Octacosanol: Refer to Venus, page 52.

Carnitine: Refer to Mars, page 63.

Chromium: Corn oil, brewer's yeast, clams, whole grain cereals.

Sulphur: Fish, eggs, cabbage, meat, asparagus, brussels sprouts, raw celery, cauliflower, onions, radishes, dried peas, cocoa, almonds, walnuts, rye, mustard, dry lentils, hard cheese, lean beef, lobsters, mustard greens, clams, dried beans, peanuts, whole wheat, spinach, barley; dried foods (prunes, raisins). Foods high in protein are also high in sulphur, for it is contained in several of the amino acids or forms of protein which are absolutely essential to human welfare.

Lecithin: Melon seeds, sunflower seeds, cereal seeds, cold pressed vegetable oils, and egg yolks.

Vitamin and Mineral Functions

Vitamin B-5: Refer to the Sun, page 24.

Vitamin B-12, B-15, Niacin, Co-enzyme Q-10: Refer to the Sun, pages 24, 25.

Vitamin B-2, B-6: Refer to the Moon, page 37.

Choline: Refer to Mercury, page 44.

Magnesium: Refer to Mercury, page 45.

Vitamin E: Refer to Venus, pages 51, 52.

Zinc, Biotin, Inositol, Vitamin F, Octacosanol: Refer to Venus, pages 55, 56.

Carnitine: Refer to Mars, page 67.

Chromium: Glucose metabolism (energy). It plays a very big part in the normal functioning of the pancreas. Its function is to prolong the time before more insulin is needed, thus it increases the effectiveness of insulin.

Sulphur: Necessary for collagen formation, the structure of (formation) the living tissues of the body. It is important for the efficient working of the human body. In the body, the muscles contain about half the sulphur, while bones and skin contain most of the rest. Sulphur foods stimulate the liver and promote the flow of bile.

Lecithin: It is an important substance to have in the diet so the body can be protected against accumulations of cholesterol. When lecithin is used properly it prevents an accumulation of cholesterol in your the vessels or bladder. In natural foods, lecithin is an emulsifying agent for the cholesterol. When the cholesterol tends to lump together, the lecithin breaks it up, mixes with it and keeps it finely divided so that it can circulate throughout the body as a perfectly stable emulsion that will not solidify or congeal. Note: Hydrogenated fats (the shortenings used in pastry and for frying) do not contain lecithin, for it has been destroyed in the hydrogenation process.

Vitamin and Mineral Deficiency Symptoms

Vitamin B-5, B-12: Refer to the Sun, page 32.

Vitamins B-15, Niacin, Co-enzyme Q-10: Refer to the Sun, page 32.

Vitamin B-2, B-6: Refer to the Moon, page 39.

Choline, Magnesium: Refer to Mercury, page 43, 44.

Vitamin E, Zinc: Refer to Venus, pages 56, 57.

Biotin, Inositol, Vitamin F, Octacosanol: Refer to Venus, page 57.

Carnitine: Refer to Mars, page 72.

Chromium: Atherosclerosis, glucose intolerance in diabetes and hypoglycemia.

Sulphur: Blood and skin diseases, eruptions, pimples, arthritis and psoriasis.

Lecithin: Lecithin is made in the liver, provided certain ingredients are present there. Choline and Vitamin F (the unsaturated fatty acids) must be present for the liver to make lecithin. When the cholesterol is not emulsified, it deposits on artery walls and there is nothing to keep the cholesterol from moving along through the blood stream; it cakes and gathers in lumps, and results in health problems - weight gain, hepatitis or a heart attach could occur.

Vitamin and Mineral Therapeutic Applications

Vitamin B-5, B-12, B-15, Niacin, Co-enzyme Q-10: Refer to the Sun, pages 34, 35.

Vitamin B-2, B-6: Refer to the Moon, page 41.

Choline, Magnesium: Refer to Mercury, page 47.

Vitamin E, Zinc, Biotin, Inositol, Vitamin F, Octacosanol: Refer to Venus, pages 58, 59.

Carnitine: Refer to Mars, page 72.

Chromium: Diabetes, hypoglycemia.

Sulphur: Helps eliminate wastes, blood and skin diseases, eruptions, pimples, psoriasis, eczema, dermatitis (as an ointment) and rheumatism. Foods containing sulphur aid in reducing. Sulphur baths are good for arthritis as they help to increase sulphur in the blood. The cystine (a form of protein) content of the fingernails increases after sulphur bath. It takes away pain.

Lecithin: Helps obesity, the heart and the liver.

Jupiter

Jupiter governs the liver, the fats and glycogen, which are stored as fuel. The arterial system of the body is ruled by Jupiter. The manufacture and secretion of insulin by the pancreas gland is influenced by Jupiter aspects. Bile is formed by the liver cells and conveys from the body waste products of the liver's activity. When Jupiter is afflicted, cholesterol and/or liver problems may develop.

When the insulin supply is abundant, such fats find their way into the blood stream and are quickly stored. Unless thyroxin and adrenalin are as abundant in proportion, this stored fat is not called upon as fuel, but continues to be stored. There is a need to increase the activity of the thyroid gland, as thyroxine enables the body to burn its excess fuel. When exercise is taken to consume excess fat, the diet should contain some starch or sugar, as fat can only burn in the presence of sugar! (Keep that in mind when on a weight-loss diet.) Absolute elimination of starch and sugar from the diet while engaging in strenuous exercise causes the fat to smolder and fill the blood with fatty acids!

Overeating, or the eating of rich foods, strains the insulin supply. When the insulin supply is exhausted, sugar can no longer be transformed into glycogen and stored. It is not transformed into fat. Instead it remains in the blood as simple sugar which being soluble is washed out of the body and lost. (There is too much insulin in proportion to adrenalin and thyroxine.) Note: Overexertion and emotional excitement could make matters worse. The preceding conditions could lead to a diabetic or hypoglycemic problem.

Insulin tries to get rid of the overtaxing burden of fat in the blood due to overeating or eating rich foods out of proportion to the amount of exercise taken. In the effort to rid the blood of fuel which cannot be burned, irritated spots are found as a convenient dumping ground and thus a fatty tumor develops. Tumors indicate an acid, or a toxic blood stream. When the blood stream is thus loaded with toxins (more fat than can be burned), diabetic and other fatty acids are liberated in the blood stream and acidosis could result.

Thus when Jupiter is afflicted in the horoscope the body may have difficulty handling fats, starches, sugars and fructose. Avoid foods rich in fat, i.e., butter, creams, gravies, sauces, oils, olives, avocados, all nuts (especially pecans, pine, macadamia, English walnuts), cheese, butternuts, egg yolks, coconut, highly rich spicy and seasoned (condiments, mustards) foods. Do not over eat! Watch carbohydrate intake too! Avoid cane sugar. Garlic reduces cholesterol. Fats such as that of meat, butter, olive oil, oils of corn and wheat (wheat germ oil, and flakes, avocados, fish liver oils, raw and unprocessed seeds and nuts especially sunflower seeds) are stored as fats, and thus become part of the body tissue. But they are chiefly used as fuel reserves for the production of energy. They are important for good health. However, when Jupiter is discordant in the horoscope, the body may be unable to handle or store them properly; vitamin supplements will aid in their proper digestion. Cysts and growths can occur when Jupiter is afflicted, especially if the health is neglected through incorrect dietary habits and a lack of vitamin and mineral supplements.

Do not buy anything that has been ``hydrogenated.'' Read labels and avoid buying solid shortenings, margarine, commercial peanut butter, crackers, prepared mixes, noodles, roasted and salted nuts, popcorn, fried foods, potato chips, corn chips, pretzels, french fries and doughnuts.

Fat (ruled by Jupiter) and calcium (ruled by Saturn) are lost when too much fat is eaten because it is not absorbed.

Saturn Afflicted...
Vitamins, Minerals

WHEN SATURN IS afflicted the body needs Vitamin A (Carotene), Vitamin C with Rose Hips, D-3, P (Bioflavonoids), Ultra
Bone Up, Calcium Citrate Supreme, MSM, Strontium (a trace
mineral), Glucosamine, Chondroitin, Silica (Cell Food Silica or
Vegetarian Silica capsules), Phosphorus, Magnesium, Copper,
and Selenium.

Note: Yucca is beneficial when Saturn is afflicted in the horoscope; it helps arthritis and aids the assimilation of calcium.
When Saturn is discordant, fluorine and silica are needed for
teeth and bone. Fluorine food sources: cabbage, asparagus, cauliflower, potatoes. Silica food sources: barley, oats (oatmeal), cabbage, onions. Trace minerals are supplements that are beneficial
for the body, especially when Saturn is afflicted in the horoscope.

Vitamin and Mineral Food Sources

Vitamin A: Refer to the Sun, page 24.

Vitamin D, Calcium, Phosphorus, Magnesium: Refer to

Mercury, page 44.

Copper: Refer to Venus, page 52.

Vitamin C and P: Refer to Mars, pages 62, 63.

Selenium: All sea vegetables (kelp, agar-agar), fish, liver, yeast, whole wheat, and vegetables that grow with selenium in the soil, i.e., corn peas, lentils, wheat, nuts (especially Brazil nuts).

Vitamin and Mineral Functions

Vitamin A: Refer to the Sun, page 26.

Vitamin D: Refer to Mercury, page 45.

Calcium, Phosphorus, Magnesium: Refer to Mercury, page 45.

Copper: Refer to Venus, page 62.

Vitamin C: Refer to Mars, page 62.

Vitamin P: Refer to Mars, page 62.

Selenium: Vitamin E in conjunction with Selenium is needed. It is oxygen-giving and increases the anti-body production and destruction of free radicals. Key cell activation appears to be highly dependent on the presence of adequate amounts of Selenium.

Vitamin and Mineral Deficiency Symptoms

Vitamin A: Refer to the Sun, page 29.

Vitamin D, Calcium, Phosphorus, Magnesium: Refer to Mercury, page 46.

Copper: Refer to Venus, page 57.

Vitamin C: Refer to Mars, page 67.

Vitamin P: Refer to Mars, page 70.

Selenium: Blood levels are commonly lower in cancer patients than healthy individuals.

Vitamin and Mineral Therapeutic Applications

Vitamin A: Refer to the Sun, page 33.

Vitamin D, Calcium, Phosphorus, Magnesium: Refer to Mercury, page 47.

Copper: Refer to Venus, page 59.

Vitamin C and P: Refer to Mars, pages 71, 72.

Selenium: Ability to reduce cancer risk has been linked to improved immunological destruction of newly formed tumor cells. It may also improve the body's resistance to many diseases caused by viruses or bacteria. Immunologically related inflammatory diseases such as arthritis can also be defended with the help of Selenium.

Saturn

The bones, teeth, ligaments and mineral salts of the body are ruled by Saturn. The action of the adrenal gland in the manufacture and secretion of adrenal (also see Mars) is influenced by Saturn aspects. Also, one hormone of the front pituitary gland is influenced by Saturn. The spleen (also see Sun) is influenced by Saturn because the spleen is the storage battery of the vital electric energy (the Sun). When Saturn is afflicted in the horoscope, the spleen is unable to get and hold reserve energy.

When Saturn is afflicted there is a lack of proper elements in the food, lack of assimilative ability and, through inadequate adrenalin, lack of ability to draw on the emergency fuel supply. Saturn is negative and subtle in its influence. It tends to the accumulations of toxins in the blood and to various chronic and wasting diseases (AIDS, cancer) which persist because of lack of vigor and energy to remove their cause. Atrophy, tuberculosis, arthritis, rheumatism, constipation, pneumonia, colds, flu and stones (kidney, gall) are types of afflictions which are characteristic of Saturn. Saturn rules the growth hormone of the front pituitary gland and when afflicted may promote abnormal growths.

When Saturn is discordant, there is a depression of the functions and deprivation of the system of its essential vitamins and minerals which causes certain elements in the blood stream (which normally enter into harmless compounds but are unable to do so while chemical imbalance lasts) to crystalize out and become deposited where they do damage, i.e., a person's weak point, the knees (Capricorn zone of the body).

When Saturn is afflicted the vitality is depleted; thus certain areas (the stomach, bowels, etc.) of the body do not have sufficient energy to do their work. When a person has a cold, the blood stream is unable to oust invading organisms. Usually negative thoughts precede a cold. When the thoughts are positive, both the electromagnetic energies and the chemical secretions are such as to resist invasion. Sedentary habits increase the chemical imbalance through lack of proper elimination (Saturn binds, such as in constipation, which it rules; therefore, avoid dairy products when Saturn is afflicted.)

The adrenalin supply is depleted through faulty elimination and food deficiency. A lack of mineral salts with which to neutralize the lactic acid and the acid toxins creates a problem. The mineral salts (also known as stabilizing salts - ruled by Saturn) share in forming bone and blood in the process of digestion, and in energy production. Acid in the blood stream is increased through dietary deficiency. If the system becomes too depleted from lack of adequate diet, from negative thinking (worry and mental exertion) or other causes, the adrenal glands become exhausted and can no longer manufacture adrenalin. This may cause the circulation to be slowed down. Thoughts of worry, fear, anxiety, depression, insecurity, unhappiness, lonesomeness, etc., cause a constriction of the arterial blood vessels and release adrenalin, which withdraws the blood from the digestive tract. Thus, whenever one is tired, negative or exposed to cold, one should not eat.

Saturn is always afflicted and involved in the diseases AIDS and cancer. Saturn, on the negative side, represents the starving or wasting away of the tissues and bones. The person loses weight and gets a haggard skeletal look (Saturn rules the skeletal part of the body). Therefore it is important to think positive, and I believe in taking the vitamins and minerals needed when Saturn is afflicted. However, when Saturn is discordant, it is possible the system is unable to properly assimilate the necessary vitamins and minerals. Proper diet may help.

Uranus Afflicted...
Vitamins, Minerals

WHEN URANUS IS afflicted, the body needs Vitamins B-1, B-6, B-12, B-15, Choline, Vitamin D (or sunlight), Calcium (Ultra Bone Up), Magnesium, Phosphorus, and Potassium.

Vitamin and Mineral Food Sources
Vitamin and Mineral Functions
Vitamin and Mineral Deficiency Symptoms
Vitamin and Mineral Therapeutic Applications

Vitamin B-1: Refer to the Sun, pages 24, 26, 30, 34.

Vitamin B-12: Refer to the Sun, pages 24, 27, 32, 34.

Vitamin B-15: Refer to the Sun, pages 24, 27, 32, 34.

Vitamin B-6, Potassium: Refer to the Moon, pages 37, 38, 39, 41.

Choline, Vitamin D, Calcium, Magnesium, Phosphorus: Refer to Mercury, pages 44, 45, 46, 47.

Uranus

Uranus rules the electrical ignition system. It's action involves the parathyroid glands. The sensitivity of the nervous system and the nerves which flow over it are influenced by Uranus. Uranus aspects increase the potential and vibratory rate of the electrical energies generated by the nerves. Thus it is involved in strokes, spasms, convulsions, all nervous disorders (breakdowns), epilepsy, paralysis, shingles, neuralgia, cerebral hemorrhage, and appendicitis. Sudden flare-ups with illness occur, often disappearing as quickly as they came. Uranus also has a pronounced influence over the action of the parathyroid glands and influences one hormone of the front pituitary gland. When Uranus is afflicted, the high tension depletes the parathyrin, which must be present to handle calcium and keep the blood stream in chemical balance. The calcium balance is disturbed, giving great sensitivity to the nerves and attracting various illnesses as mentioned previously. Therefore, it is important for the body to get calcium and other needed vitamins and minerals when Uranus is afflicted.

Neptune Afflicted...
Vitamins, Minerals

WHEN NEPTUNE IS afflicted the body needs Vitamins B-1, B-2, B-6, B-12 (or Cracked Cell Chlorella if an allergy to B-12 exists), Biotin, Choline, Folic Acid, Niacin (no flush), Paba, Vitamin C with Rose Hips), Vitamin D-3, Vitamin P (Bioflavonoids), Calcium Citrate Supreme, Ultra Bone Up, Phosphorus, Charcoal (for gas), Ginger capsules (for gas, aids digestion), and Brewer's Yeast.

Note: When Neptune is afflicted the body needs to be detoxed (refer to Part One/Chapter Two, page 9) of the many poisons (Neptune rules poisons) that have accumulated in the system.

When there is a yeast problem (candida albicans), brewer's yeast should not be taken; perhaps, a food substitute which does not contain, or feed, yeast would be the best choice.

Thiotic Acid (Thiox), supposedly can oxidize serious poisons such as Mercury toxemia, and destroy angel mushroom poisoning. It is also supposed to be helpful in alcoholism and narcotic addition as well as various poisonings. It may be an aid to those who want to quit smoking. Neptune rules nicotine, drugs (narcotic and patent medicine) and alcohol.

Vitamin and Mineral Food Sources
Vitamin and Mineral Functions
Vitamin and Mineral Deficiency Symptons
Vitamin and Mineral Therapeutic Applications

Vitamin B-1: Refer to the Sun, pages 24, 26, 30, 34.

Vitamin B-12: Refer to the Sun, pages 24, 27, 32, 34.

Folic Acid, Niacin: Refer to the Sun, pages, 25, 27, 32, 34.

Vitamin B-2, B-6: Refer to the Moon, pages 37, 38, 39, 41.

Choline, Vitamin D, Calcium, Phosphorus: Refer to Mercury, pages 43, 44, 45, 46, 47.

Biotin: Refer to Venus, pages 52, 55, 57, 59.

PABA: Refer to Mars, pages 62, 64, 67, 71.

Vitamin C: Refer to Mars, pages 62, 64, 67, 71.

Vitamin P: Refer to Mars, pages 62, 66, 70, 72.

Pancreatin: Refer to Mars, pages 63, 66, 70, 72.

Neptune

Neptune is involved with the action of the parathyroid glands, thus the nervous system becomes sensitive. The hormone of the pineal gland is influenced by Neptune. This hormone suppresses and counteracts the action of cortin (the strongest chemical with which the body fights toxins and poisons). The excessive negative condition thus induced tends to the accumulation of toxins. Neptune is the poisoner (Neptune rules poisons taken internally, or by snake or spider bite, poison ivy, asphyxiation, or food toxins) and because it reduces the action of the cortin and also of adrenalin (ruled by Mars), the poisons cannot be eliminated from the body. The manufacturing of adrenalin is suppressed when Neptune is afflicted (it also combats infections and toxins). Neptune attracts the formation of pus, invasion of bacteria (moist pockets), fungus, parasites, worms, wax in ears and mosit-wasting diseases. When Neptune is afflicted in the horoscope, be careful of giving in to the use of narcotics, opiates and alcohol. The desire may be to escape into another world where everything is as desired in the world of the unreal-never-never land. And when "high" the only desire is to continue escaping and daydreaming.

When Neptune is afflicted in the horoscope, the low output of cortin (hormone) results in the incomplete metabolism of protein foods with an accumulation of toxins. Therefore, less protein is needed; however, if hypoglycemic, more protein is needed. (Neptune is involved in hypoglycemia.) Neptune rules fainting and dizziness, and one may feel lazy, tired, sleepy, and thus take naps or procrastinate; this indicates the probability of poisons in the system. Detoxify. Avoid gas-forming foods. (Usually there is a lot of gas in the system when Neptune is afflicted).

The ability of the parathyroid glands to handle calcium is reduced when Neptune is discordant in the horoscope. The diet should be such as to give the blood stream an alkaline reaction to assist it and neutralize the toxic condition. Usually, loss of memory is coincidental with toxic poisoning. Neptune is also involved with the diseases AIDS, cancer and Alzheimer's.

When Neptune is afflicted the likelihood is great for a yeast infection. Also, when when Neptune is discordant, doctors could give a wrong diagnosis. However, a person with candida albicans (yeast infection) needs to change the diet.

Candida Symptoms

Cravings for sugar, bread or alcoholic beverages; frequent headaches, anxiety, confusion, loss of memory, severe depression, lack of energy, disorientation, insomnia or the opposite, impotence, vaginal infection, rectal itching, jock itch, recurrent bladder infections, chronic diarrhea, constipation, menstrual irregularity and severe cramps, bloating and gas, swelling of joints, fungal infections, athlete's foot, digestive disorder, abdominal pain, heartburn, chest pain, muscular weakness, blurred vision, recurrent sore throat, nasal congestion, persistent cough, rash, or blister in mouth, or fluid in the ears.

Foods That Help Eliminate Yeast, Strengthen Immune System

Garlic, onions, cabbage, ginger root, broccoli, barley, turnips, kale, oats, wheat germ, yogurt, olive oil, lobster, shrimp, scallops, and Brazil nuts.

When vitamins are purchased make sure they are yeast and sugar free. In addition to the vitamins listed for what the body needs when Neptune is afflicted, there are others that are needed when one has candida: Vitamin A, B-3, B-5, Bee Pollen, Magnesium, Iron, Zinc, Selenium, Evening Primrose Oil, Vitamin E, amino acids, odorless garlic capsules.

Foods to Avoid When One Has Candida

Avoid sugar products including honey, maple syrup, molasses, and maple, date and turbinado sugar. Candida and also cancer cells multiply when fed sugar products. Read labels on all packaged and frozen foods. These forms of sugar are all bad: maltose, fructose, lactose, glycogen, galactose, sorbital, glucose, mannitol, sucrose, monosaccharide, and polysaccharide, brown sugar, and raw sugar.

Do not eat any fruits (other than grapefruit) because they contain fructose. Avoid junk foods, especially those that contain food coloring, additives, and hydrogenated or partially hydrogenated vegetable oil. Do not eat processed food, including nuts. Eat unprocessed nuts, seeds and oils. However, many people with Candida are allergic to nuts, molds, yeasts - therefore, avoid mushrooms, truffles, leftovers unless properly refrigerated (freeze instead), cheese (especially moldy ones, i.e. roquefort) and prepared foods containing cheese; avoid sour milk products, tofu; liqueur (including wine, beer, liqueurs and fermented beverages, e.g. cider, root beer); avoid breads, pastries and bakery products containing yeast; avoid malt products (candy, cereal, malted drinks); avoid foods containing vinegar (ketchup, pickles, sauerkraut, salad dressings, mayonnaise, marinated vegetables, relishes, green olives, horseradish); avoid condiments (mustard, accent, MSG - monosodium glutamate, mince meat, curry and steak, barbecue, shrimp, chili, tamari, and soy sauces); avoid coffee and tea (including herbal teas); avoid canned, processed and fast foods (including sausages, hot dogs, corned beef, pickled tongue, pastrami, turkey, chicken); avoid dried and candied fruits (dates, figs, raisins, prunes, apricots, pineapples); avoid melons (cantaloupe, honeydew, watermelon); avoid fruit juices either canned, bottled or frozen (except freshly prepared grapefruit juice).

Foods That Can Be Eaten When One Has Candida

These foods help strengthen the immune system: Eggs, fish (not breaded), salmon, tuna, cod, sardines, mackerel; seafood (shrimp, lobster, crab); chicken, turkey, cornish hens, wild game; lamb, pork and lean cut beef; vegetables high in fiber content and low in carbohydrates such as asparagus, cabbage, beets, Brussels sprouts, carrots, broccoli, cauliflower, eggplant, celery, cucumbers, green pepper, okra, onions, parsley, radishes, string beans, tomatoes, soybeans, lettuce (all types) and greens - dandelion, beet, turnip, collard, kale, spinach and mustard.

Neptune Afflicted...Vitamins, Minerals

Pluto Afflicted...
Vitamins, Minerals

WHEN PLUTO IS afflicted the body needs Vitamin A (Carotene), Vitamins B-2, B-5, B-6, B-12, Biotin, Folic Acid (B-9), Potassium, Niacin (no flush), PABA, Vitamin C with Rose Hips, Vitamin D-3, Vitamin P (Bioflavonoids), Calcium Citrate Supreme, Ultra Bone Up, Iron, Manganese, Zinc, Pancreatin (quadruple strength), and Selenium. Note: Thiotic Acid may be good for allergies (Pluto afflicted) and Chemical (Pluto) Hypersensitivity Syndrome.

Vitamin and Mineral Food Sources
Vitamin and Mineral Functions
Vitamin and Mineral Deficiency Symptoms
Vitamin and Mineral Therapeutic Applications

Manganese, Vitamin A: Refer to the Sun, pages 24, 26, 29, 33.

Vitamin B-5, B-12, B-15, Folic Acid, Niacin: Refer to the Sun, pages 24, 25, 27, 32, 34.

Vitamin B-2, B-6, Potassium: Refer to the Moon, pages 37, 38, 39, 41.

Vitamin D, Calcium: Refer to Mercury, pages 44, 45, 46, 47.

Zinc, Biotin: Refer to Venus, pages 52, 55, 57, 59.

PABA: Refer to Mars, pages 62, 64, 67, 71.

Vitamin C: Refer to Mars, pages 62, 64, 67, 71.

Vitamin P, Iron: Refer to Mars, pages 62, 63, 66, 70, 72.

Pancreatin: Refer to Mars, pages 63, 66, 70, 72.

Selenium: Refer to Saturn, page 86, 87.

Pluto

Pluto rules four endocrine glands: the hormone of the pineal gland, one hormone of the front pituitary, the cortin hormone of the adrenal cortex and secretions of the parathyroid glands. When the pineal secretion (rather than cortin) is increased (Pluto afflicted), the same negative condition and susceptibility to toxic poisons brought about by the influence of Neptune take place.

When Pluto is afflicted the body's manufacture of adrenalin and cortin (the strongest chemical with which the body fights toxins and infections) is suppressed. The low output of cortin hormone results in the incomplete metabolism of protein foods with an accumulation of toxic build-up. Pluto afflicted reduces the ability of the parathyroid glands to handle calcium. Note: Pluto is involved in the disease AIDS.

Daily Dosage...Vitamins and Minerals... Brand Names, Units

Twin Lab Brand
  B-1 Caps, 100 mg.
  B-2 Caps, 100 mg.
  B-5 Caps, 100 mg.
  B-6 Caps, 500 mg.
  Manganese caps, 10 mg.
  L. Carnitine caps, 250 mg.
  Magnesium caps, 400 mg.
  Carotene (A) caps, 25,000 I.U.
  Niacin caps, (B-3), 100 mg.
  Chline & Inositol Caps, 500 mg.
  Paba caps, 500 mg.
  Chromium Caps (Glucose Tolerance Factor tablets), 200
    mcg.
  Potassium caps, 99 mg.
  Folic Acid caps, 800 mg.
  Zinc caps, 50 mg.
  Germanium tablets, 25 mg.
  Vitamin P (Bioflavonoids)
  Betaine Hydrochloric
  Octacosanol
  Pancreatin
Schiff Brand
  Vitamin C (Rose Hips), 500 mg.
Jarrow Brand
  Vitamin D-3

Bone Up
Coenzyme Q-10

Solgar Brand
Acidophilus caps
Liverall caps, 7 and 1/2 grain
B-12 caps, 500 mcg.
Selenium tablets, 50 mcg.
Biotin tablets, 300 mg.
Boron caps, 3 mg.
L. Arginine, 500 mg.
Lecithin Softgels, 260 mg.

Rhondell Brand
Phosphorus tablets, 100 mg.

French Riviera Brand
Bee Pollen, 500 mg.

The Ion Performance Line
Colon "8" caplets

Nutri-dyn Brand
Trace Min. tablets (Multi-minerals with Vitamins D, B-6,
Glutamic Acid HCI, Zinc, Manganese, Potassium)

Udo's Oil Blend (Evening Primrose Oil, Flax Oil—Omega 3,
6, 9)

Life Time Brand
Cracked Cell Chlorella (Iron, Vitamins A and B-2, Chlorophyll)

Kal Brand
Sod-3

Nature's Plus Brand
Chlorophyll caps 100 mg.
Co-enzyme Q-10 softgels, 30 mg.
Vitamin F caps, 1000 mg.

Iron tablets, (Amino Acid Chelated), Vegetarian, 40 mg.

Himalaya Brand

Liver Care

Bladder Care

Kidney Care

Nature's Way....Herb Capsules

Cayenne, 450 mg.

Fenugreek seed, 610 mg.

Chickweed, 385 mg.

Golden Seal, 400 mg.

Comfrey Pepsin (comfrey root 490 mg., Pepsin 100 mg.)

HIGL (for hypoglycemia) 480 mg.

Dandelion root, 510 mg.

Red Clover blossoms, 430 mg.

Echinacea, 380 mg.

Thisilyn, 330 mg.

Yucca stalk, 490 mg.

Table B - Afflicted Planets

Name_____

Find afflicted planet and write below the dates discorandantly
aspected. Look up that planet on its page in Lynne Palmer's *As-
tro-Guide to Nutrition and Vitamins* to identify that planet's vitamin and mineral food sources, function, deficiency symptoms
and therapeutic applications.

Sun Afflicted_____

Moon Afflicted_____

Mercury Afflicted_____

Venus Afflicted_____

Mars Afflicted_____

Jupiter Afflicted_____

Saturn Afflicted_____

Uranus Afflicted_____

Neptune Afflicted_____

Pluto Afflicted_____

Marla

October 27, 1962, 11:49 AM EST, 84W58 34N46
Complete Secondary Progressions for 3 Years
MC progressed by solar arc. One degree orbs used for all aspects.
Natal planets are enclosed in parentheses.
Applying aspects are in upper case.
Separating aspects are in lower case.
- - - indicates the event occurs outside the range of the report.
// denotes a NN or SS parallel aspect;
# denotes a NS or SN parallel aspect.

January 1, 1991

House	Planet	Longitude	Declination
11	Sun	Sag 2 7	20 35 S
10	Moon	Sco 5 18	8 31 S
11	Mercury	Sag 1 49	21 2 S
10	Venus	Sco 13 43R	16 57 S
8	Mars	Leo 19 19	17 9 N
2	Jupiter	Pis 3 59	11 11 S
1	Saturn	Aqu 6 30	19 23 S
8	Uranus	Vir 5 11	10 19 N
10	Neptune	Sco 13 55	14 23 S
8	Pluto	Vir 12 3	19 19 N
1	ASC	Aqu 4 17	19 12 S
11	MC	Sco 22 59	18 31 S

Aspects Forming During the Coming Year

Enter	Aspect	Exact	Leave
1 Jan 91	Merc SQR (Jupi)	8/20/92	4/08/92
13 Jul 91	MC SSX (Moon)	7/08/92	7/04/93
5 Aug 91	Jupi SSX (Satn)	—	—
6 Aug 91	MC = (Mars)	—	—
13 Aug 91	Merc SSX (Sun)	4/01/92	11/19/92
2 Sep 91	MC SSX (MC)	8/27/92	8/23/93
2 Sep 91	Sun SSX (Sun)	8/27/92	8/23/93
13 Oct 91	Merc SQR Jupi	6/15/92	2/16/93
9 Nov 91	MC = (Satn)	—	—
11 Dec 91	Sun SQR Jupi	1/10/93	—

Aspects in Orb

Aspect	Exact	Leave	Aspect	Exact	Leave
Sun SSQ (Merc)	---	10/31/91	Sat # Plu	10/07/93	---
Sun SQR (Jup)	9/13/91	9/08/92	Ur TRI (Asc)	---	---
Sun # (Mars)	---	6/09/91	Ur # (MC)	---	---
Sun // (Sat)	---	10/07/91	Plu SXT (Nep)	---	---
Merc SSQ (Merc)	2/01/91	9/20/91	Plu # (Sat)	---	---
Ven CON (Nep)	12/01/93	---	Plu // (Mars)	---	---
Mars SQQ (Asc)	2/01/93	---	Asc SQR (Sun)	---	5/31/91
Jup TRI (Sun)	---	---	Asc CON (Sat)	8/12/91	5/30/92
Jup OPP (Ur)	---	---	Asc QCX (Ur)	2/07/91	11/29/91
Jup SXT (Asc)	---	---	Asc SSX (ASC)	7/22/91	5/10/92
Jup # (Ur)	---	---	Asc # (Mars)	---	9/16/92
Sat # (Mars)	---	---	Asc # (Plu)	---	10/16/93
Sat # (Plu)	11/25/93	---	ASC // (Sat)	---	7/02/92
Ur QCX (Sat)	---	---	MC # (Plu)	---	---
Sun CON Merc	7/09/91	7/19/93	Sat [ASC	---	10/14/93
Sun // Merc	---	8/31/93	Sat [MC	---	---
Ven CON Nep	---	5/18/93	Ur QCX ASC	9/27/91	7/18/92
Ven # Mars	---	---	Plu # ASC	---	10/13/93
Jup SSX Asc	---	8/12/91	Plu # MC	---	---
Jup # Ur	---	---	Asc // MC	3/18/92	12/27/93

Lunar Aspects

Aspect	Exact	Aspect	Exact
6 Feb 91	SQR Saturn	17 Aug 91	CON (Neptune)
21 Mar 91	SQR (Mars)	5 Sep 91	CON Venus
6 Apr 91	// (MC) 7mo	6 Sep 91	// Jupiter 7mo
17 Jun 91	# Uranus 7mo	18 Sep 91	CON Neptune
9 Jul 91	SXT (Pluto)	27 Oct 91	// (Jupiter) 7mo
12 Jul 91	# (Uranus) 7mo	18 Dec 91	SSX (Mercury
24 Jul 91	SXT Pluto		

Lightning Source UK Ltd.
Milton Keynes UK
UKHW041214040122
396596UK00004B/1228